Epilepsy - Seizures without Triggers

Edited by Kaneez Fatima Shad

Published in London, United Kingdom

Epilepsy - Seizures without Triggers
http://dx.doi.org/10.5772/intechopen.100833
Edited by Kaneez Fatima Shad

Contributors
Shao-Wen Hung, Chia-Chi Chen, Hsiao-Yun Chen, Ying-Ching Hung, Ping-Min Huang, Chia-Yu Lin, Rhoda Olowe Taiwo, Tawfeeq Shekh-Ahmad, Tak Lap Poon, Joyce Shuk Wan Chow, Darya A. Sitovskaya, Yulia Mikhailovna M. Zabrodskaya, Olga N. Gaykova, Mikhail V. Alexandrov, Sofiia E. Cherenkova, Elena D. Bazhanova, Anastasya V. Litovchenko, Tatyana V. Sokolova, Natalya M. Paramonova, Nirmeen A. Kishk, Mai B. Belal Ahmed Mohamed Nassar, Kaneez Fatima Shad, Tushar Das

First published in London, United Kingdom, 2023 by IntechOpen
IntechOpen is the global imprint of INTECHOPEN LIMITED, registered in England and Wales, registration number: 11086078, 5 Princes Gate Court, London, SW7 2QJ, United Kingdom

British Library Cataloguing-in-Publication Data
A catalogue record for this book is available from the British Library

Additional hard and PDF copies can be obtained from orders@intechopen.com

Epilepsy - Seizures without Triggers
Edited by Kaneez Fatima Shad
p. cm.
Print ISBN 978-1-80356-599-6
Online ISBN 978-1-80356-600-9
eBook (PDF) ISBN 978-1-80356-601-6

Meet the editor

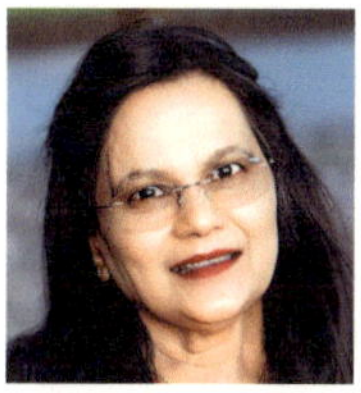

Professor Kaneez Fatima Shad, an Australian neuroscientist with a medical background, received her Ph.D. in 1994 from the Faculty of Medicine, UNSW, Australia, followed by post-doctoral research at the Allegheny University of Health Sciences, Philadelphia, USA. She has taught medical and biological sciences at various universities in Australia, USA, UAE, Bahrain, Pakistan, and Brunei. During this period, she has been engaged in research, obtaining local and international grants totaling over 3.5 million USD and translating them into products such as rapid diagnostic tests for stroke and other vascular disorders such as schizophrenia. She has published over 60 articles in refereed journals, edited nine books, written 10 book chapters, presented at over 85 international conferences, and mentored 34 postgraduate students. She is a mentor and a protocol development specialist. For further information, see the home page www.fatimashad.com and https://scholar.google.com/citations?user=eCibXd8AAAAJ&hl=en

Contents

Preface

Epilepsy is one of the most widespread neurological disorders. It has high morbidity and mortality rates and affects around 50 million people globally. Epileptic seizures have psychosocial consequences for patients and can result in several cognitive impairments. The occurrence of epilepsy is a self-facilitated pathological process triggered by the initial brain damage, ultimately leading to the loss of excitatory and inhibitory neurons in specific areas of the brain. Decades of research have failed to fully illuminate its etiology, and preventive or disease-modifying therapies are still lacking. New insights into the mechanisms of epilepsy are required to create effective treatments.

Epilepsy - Seizures without Triggers contains six distinct and enlightening chapters addressing epileptic seizures from various perspectives. Reading the first two chapters on the basic aspects makes one understand how epilepsy is related to the conditions like ferroptosis and neuroinflammation. The role of Fenton and Haber Weiss reaction in ferroptosis and epilepsy is described in the first chapter. Later chapters examine the role of epileptic focus in drug-resistant epilepsy and consider how microglia grow into an over-activated form and induce significant and highly detrimental neurotoxic factors that play a significant role in epileptogenesis.

The medical aspects section of the book begins by describing psychogenic non-epileptic seizures, followed by the management of cryptogenic epilepsy. Last but not least, readers will be captivated by the chapter on the development of pediatric epilepsy in Sub-Saharan Africa, including West Africa, due to onchocerciasis (river blindness).

Production of this book would not have been possible without the contributions of the experts in the field and the continuous hard work of IntechOpen's Author Service Manager Marina Dušević. I hope those who read it will benefit from a better understanding of the various aspects of epilepsy. Finally, I would like to emphasize that this book is meant for a broad range of readers, including people with an interest in epilepsy, undergraduate and graduate students, researchers, teachers, medical professionals, and neurological experts.

Kaneez Fatima Shad
Life Sciences,
University of Technology Sydney,
Ultimo, Australia

Section 1

Essentials of Epilepsy

Chapter 1

Introductory Chapter: Role of Fenton and Haber-Weiss Reaction in Epilepsy

Kaneez Fatima Shad and Tushar Kanti Das

1. Introduction

Epilepsy is one of the most widespread brain diseases worldwide. It has high morbidity and mortality rates and affects around 70 million people globally. Epileptic seizures have several cognitive impairments and psychosocial consequences in patients. The occurrence of epilepsy is a self-facilitated pathological process triggered by the initial brain damage, ultimately leading to the loss of excitatory and inhibitory neurons in specific areas of the brain. Decades of research failed to fully illuminate its etiology, whereas preventive or disease-modifying therapies are still missing. New insights into the mechanisms of epilepsy are required to create the effective treatments.

Oxidative stress is a contributing factor to the onset and evolution of epilepsy. The association between free radical production and oxidative stress is regarded as a possible mechanism involved in epileptogenesis.

In the following pages of this chapter, we will be looking at the role of Fenton and Haber-Weiss reaction in triggering epilepsy leading to the loss of excitatory and inhibitory neurons in specific regions of the brain.

Brain is the most vulnerable organ to oxidative stress due to its high oxygen intake and reduced antioxidative protection [1]. Excessive oxidative stress is one of the main causes of epileptic seizures. The association between free radical production and oxidative stress is regarded as a possible mechanism involved in epileptogenic seizures [2, 3].

The Fenton and Haber-Weiss reaction has a significant role in the generation of free radicals such as superoxide and highly toxic hydroxyl ions causing epileptic episodes [4, 5].

In this chapter, we discussed the role of the Fenton reaction and Haber-Weiss reaction in ferroptosis and epilepsy that provide a new direction for understanding the underlying mechanisms of epilepsy leading to new therapeutic targets.

2. Chemistry of Fenton and Haber-Weiss reaction

H.J. Fenton first described the oxidation of tartaric acid by hydrogen peroxide in the presence of ferrous irons, and then, it is known as the Fenton reaction [6, 7]. Fenton reaction can be carried out by two pathways: radical and non-radical systems for Fenton reaction [8, 9].

2.1 Radical system for Fenton reaction

Hydroxyl radical ($OH^{\cdot}$) is mainly produced by the reaction between ferrous iron and hydrogen peroxide. The Fenton reaction requires a set of conditions such as pH, temperature, concentration of hydrogen peroxide, and iron [10].

The Fenton reaction needs acidic conditions (pH = 3–4) for its catalytic activities, which gradually decreases due to the precipitation of iron as Fe $(OH)_3$ and the degradation of H_2O_2 into O_2 and H_2O [8, 11]. At the higher temperature, the rate of the reaction is increased, along with the increased decomposition rate of hydrogen peroxide [10, 12]. Increasing the concentration of Fe^{2+} leads to higher reaction rates until it reaches a certain concentration above which all rate increases appear to be marginal [13]. An adequate concentration of H_2O_2 is also needed for the reaction. Moreover, the Haber-Weiss reaction was first proposed by F. Haber and J J Weiss in 1932. Fe^{3+} is reduced to Fe^{2+} through the reaction with superoxide ($O_2^{\cdot -}$) and H_2O_2. Finally, $OH^{\cdot}$, OH^{-}, and oxygen are produced:

$$\begin{aligned} Fe^{2+} + H_2O_2 &\longrightarrow Fe^{3+} + OH + OH^{-} \text{ [Fenton reaction]} \\ OH + H_2O_2 &\longrightarrow O_2^{-} + H^{+} + H_2O \\ O_2^{-} + H_2O_2 &\xrightarrow{Fe^{3+}/Fe^{2+}} OH + OH^{-} + O_2 \text{ [Haber-Weiss reaction]} \end{aligned} \tag{1}$$

Due to the presence of multivalency of iron, iron can react with H_2O_2 by one- or two-electron transfer. Several studies indicate that as a classical Fenton reaction, Fe^{2+} reacts with H_2O_2 by the outer sphere electron transfer with no direct bonding interactions between the electron donor and the acceptor [8]. Other studies also indicate that metal-centered Fenton reaction occurs by the direct bonding between iron and H_2O_2 by inner sphere electron transfer mechanisms. This interaction could produce a metal-peroxo complex, Fe (II)HOO, which may react further to generate either HO· radicals (one-electron oxidant) or Fe (IV)O (two-electron oxidant) (**Figure 1**).

2.2 Non-radical system for Fenton reaction

Non-radical Fenton reaction begins with the reversible reaction between Fe^{2+} and H_2O_2. [Fe^{2+}. H_2O_2], [FeO^{2+}], and $[FeOFe]^{5+}$ are the most important intermediate products of this reaction. The reaction is carried out either through oxidation or reduction reaction of iron ions and addition or subtraction of H_2O_2 reaction [8, 9]. The overall reaction is represented in **Figure 2**.

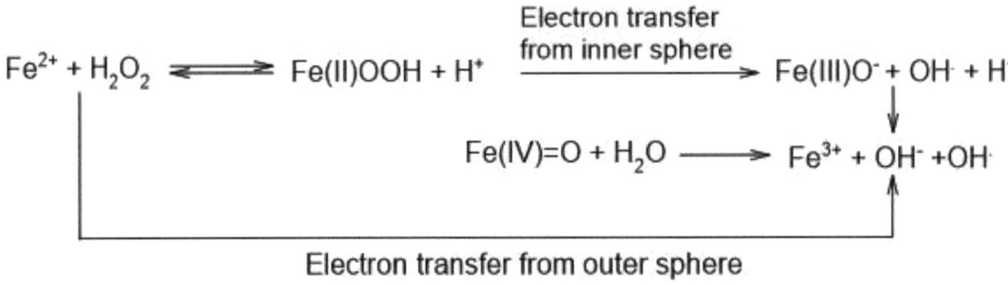

Figure 1.
The reaction mechanism of the classical and metal-centered Fenton reaction [8].

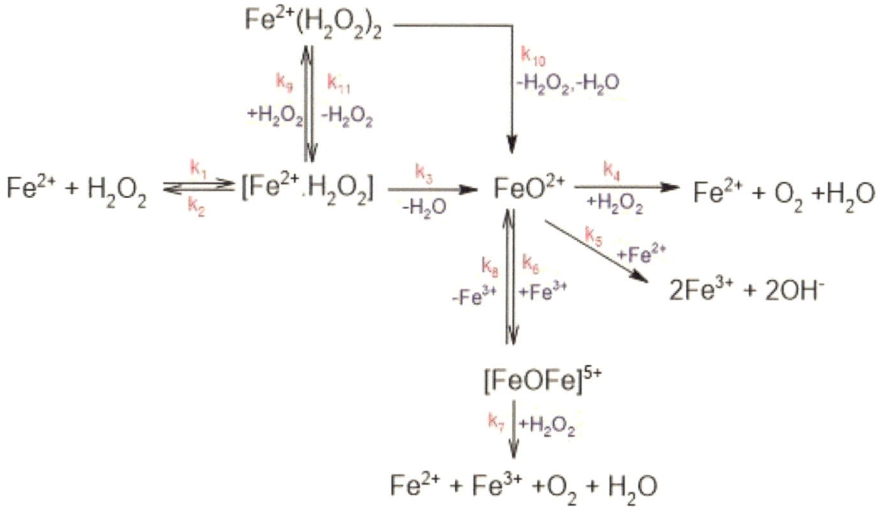

Figure 2.
Reaction mechanism of non-radical Fenton reaction [8, 9].

In addition, the Fenton reaction is catalyzed by several transition metals such as iron, zinc, copper, cobalt, manganese [14] The overall reaction is represented as follows:

$$Mn^{+} + H_2O_2 = Mn^{+} + OH^{-} + OH \quad (2)$$

The capacity of metal ions to induce epilepsy is well known. The concentration of Fe^{2+}, Zn^{2+}, Cu^{2+}, and CO^{2+} are higher in the epileptic human brain compared with the healthy brain. The abnormal levels of trace metals may be epileptogenic, and they enhance excitatory synaptic mechanisms and reduce inhibitory processes. These metal ions also produce higher concentrations of hydroxyl radicals by the Fenton and Haber-Weiss reaction in epilepsy [5, 15, 16].

3. Fenton and Haber-Weiss reaction in epilepsy

Reactive oxygen species (ROS) play a major role in epilepsy [2, 16]. ROS is generated by many cellular processes such as mitochondrial metabolism, cellular respiration, metabolism of organic matter through a redox reaction, and tissue homeostasis. High-reactive hydroxyl radical is produced by the Fenton and Haber-Weiss reaction in the presence of suitable transition metal. Iron is abundant in the epileptic brain and is involved in the formation of hydroxyl radicals [5, 15].

In 2012, Dixon et al. first discovered iron-dependent cell death by the accumulation of iron-dependent free radicals, and this process is known as "ferroptosis" [17]. Therefore, the imbalance of ROS production is an important factor in ferroptosis. Burdened iron is a common cause of hemorrhagic post-stroke epilepsy and post-traumatic epilepsy [18, 19]. Enormous evidence suggests that a chronic epileptic animal model is created by the injection of hemoglobin or iron into the cortex of an animal [20, 21]. Higher levels of intracellular superoxide and hydroxyl radicals are found in the cerebral cortex after ferric chloride injection [22]. Other studies showed

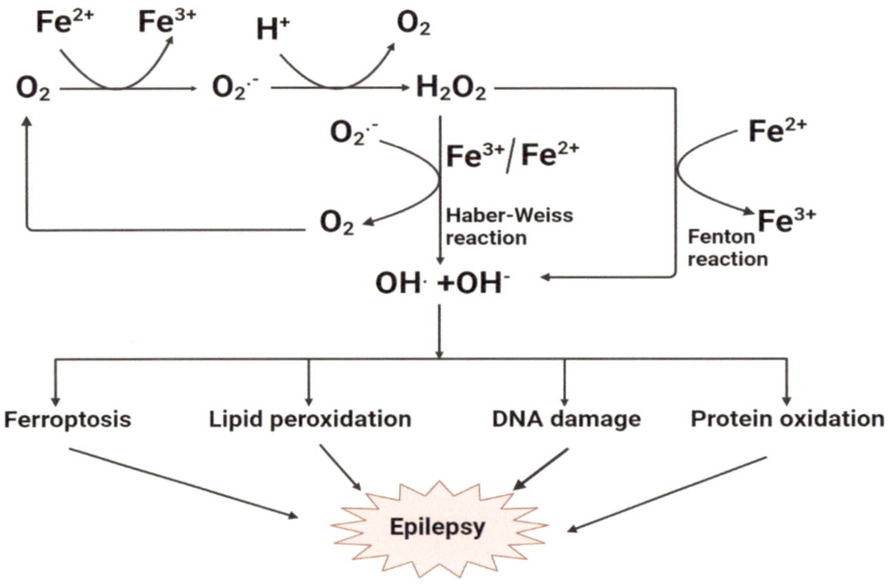

Figure 3.
The association between the Fenton and Haber-Weiss reaction and epilepsy [5, 15].

that concentrations of transferrin are markedly higher in patients with epilepsy [23]. It boosts iron intake into the cell and accelerates ferroptosis. In addition, sudden unexpected death in epilepsy is caused by cardiomyocyte ferroptosis in the heart through excess production of ROS [24]. Therefore, activation of the ferroptosis pathway is implicated in the pathogenesis of epilepsy and epileptic neuronal death. Excess iron ions generate hydroxyl radicals, which have high reactivity with proteins, lipids, and nucleic acids, leading to lipid peroxidation and promoting ferroptosis in epilepsy (**Figure 3**).

3.1 Fenton and Heber-Weiss reactions and Ferroptosis

Iron is a crucial element in cellular metabolism, energy generation, and growth in organisms. It participates in various oxidation-reduction reactions. Iron tends to be stored and transported in the Fe^{3+} form. In the blood, Fe^{3+} binds to transferrin (Tf) to form a complex which can be delivered into the cells by binding to transferrin receptor-1 (TFR1) in the cell membrane and then transported to the endosome [25]. Then, Fe^{3+} is converted to Fe^{2+} by an oxidation-reduction process with the help of six-transmembrane epithelial antigen of prostate 3 (STEAP3) and divalent metal transporter 1 (DMT1) and then released into the labile iron pool of mitochondria, lysosome, cytosol, and the nucleus [26]. Iron can also be exported by ferroprotein, an iron efflux pump in the cellular membrane, which can oxidize Fe^{2+} to Fe^{3+}. Excess Fe^{2+} reacts with H_2O_2 and produces OH^- anion and $OH^·$ radical by the Fenton reaction in ferroptosis. Moreover, the Haber-Weiss cycle showed that Fe^{3+} is reduced to Fe^{2+} through the reaction with superoxide ($O_2^·$), and Fe^{2+} reacts with H_2O_2 and forms $OH^·$, OH^-, and $Fe^{3+·}$ Thus, Fe^{2+} is conducive to the production of ROS and promotes ferroptosis [15]. Autophagy can modulate the sensitivity to ferroptosis *via* the selective autophagy of ferritin; this process is called "ferritinophagy." Nuclear receptor

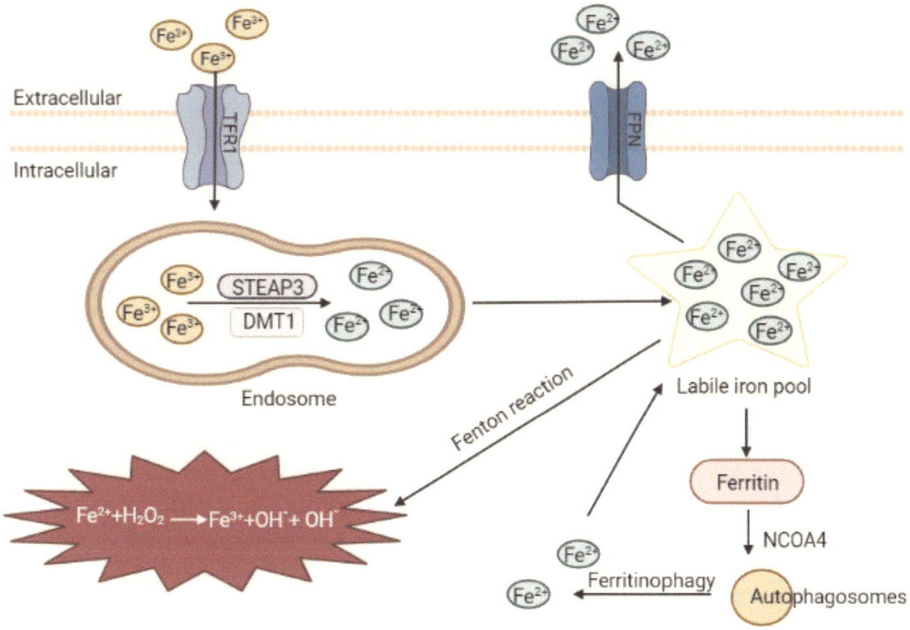

Figure 4.
Schematic representation of iron metabolism and ferroptosis associated with Fenton and Haber-Weiss reaction [15].

coactivator 4 (NCOA4) binds to ferritin and then delivers it to autophagosomes for lysosomal degradation. Fe^{2+} is released in the cell by degradation, which promotes ferroptosis (**Figure 4**).

3.2 Fenton and Haber-Weiss reaction and lipid peroxidation

Numerous lipid species are distributed in intra- or extra-cellular areas and play important roles in the energy supply and structural components of the intracellular membrane system. Cell membranes are sensitive to radical damage due to the presence of polyunsaturated fatty acids (PUFAs). Free radical oxidizes PUFAs, leading to the formation of hydroperoxides lipid and alkyl radical. This lipoperoxidation alters membrane structure, damages its fluidity integrity, and finally causes ferroptosis [27]. Due to the presence of double bonds, PUFAs are one of the most reactive substrates toward free radicals mainly hydroxyl radicals. Hydroxyl-dependent and hydroxyl-independent pathways are the main routes for the lipid peroxidation process [28]. The Fenton reaction and Haber-Weiss reaction are involved in a hydroxyl-dependent pathway, whereas Fe^{2+} accelerates hydroxyl-independent lipid peroxidation. As a result, ferroptosis also gets accelerated [5, 15, 28].

The lipid peroxidation process is initiated by the attack of hydroxyl radicals at bis-allelic positions in the fatty acid side chains, leading to generating of an alkyl radical. The radical is stabilized by the resonance with the double bond. Then, a chain reaction occurs with the extension of the damage and formation of further radical spices, and this process is known as the propagation phase. A newly formed radical reacts with oxygen and forms a peroxyl radical ($LOO^{\cdot}$), which can react with other adjacent PUFAs to form a hydroperoxide and an alkyl radical, and it causes a chain reaction and

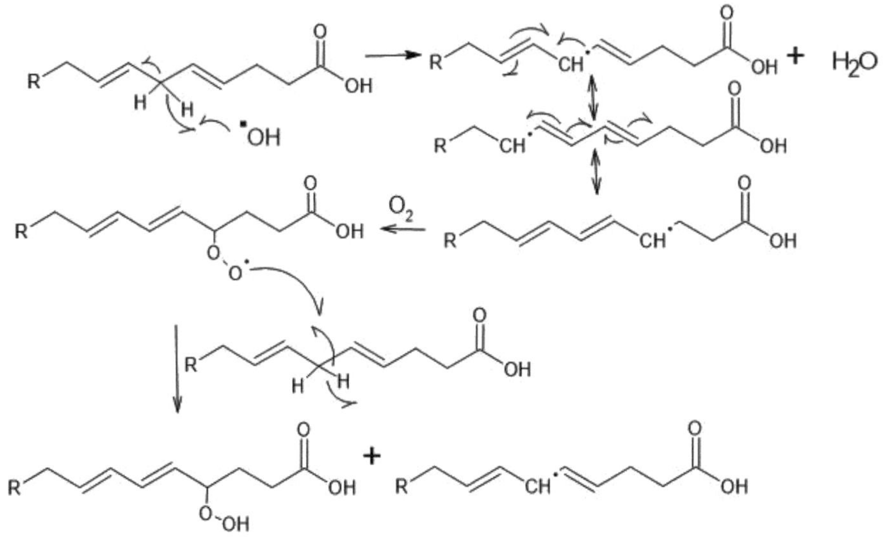

Figure 5.
Lipid peroxidation mechanism by hydroxyl radical [28].

damages more fatty acids [28]. In lipid peroxidation, the fatty acid undergoes a further reaction with oxygen and produces hydroperoxynonenal and then hydroxynonenal (**Figure 5**).

In a nutshell, in the presence of excess iron ions, lipid peroxidation forms more lipid-free radicals and serves as a trigger for ferroptosis.

3.3 Fenton and Haber-Weiss reaction and DNA damage

Mitochondrial DNA (mtDNA) is mainly susceptible to ROS due to its proximity, despite being packaged with proteins as protective covering. Its mutation can lead to a variety of diseases such as epilepsy.

In DNA, ROS reacts with nitrogenous bases and deoxyribose. This can lead to mutations, carcinogenesis, apoptosis, and necrosis. Hydroxyl radical causes direct damage to DNA, mainly by standard excision, and causes oxidative damage to the pyrimidine and purine bases. This process starts with the radical-induced abstraction of a proton from any position of the deoxyribose and can result in many products (**Figure 6**). In thymine, the abstraction of methyl hydrogen from the 5-position by the hydroxyl radical generates a resonance-stabilized carbon radical, which provides the hydroxymethylene derivative, after treatment with oxygen and followed by reduction.

3.4 Protein oxidation and Fenton Haber-Weiss reaction

Proteins are encoded by nuclear and mitochondrial DNA, which have numerous functions in the cells. Their function and regulation depend on their structures. Oxidative stress damages their structural integrity, causes loss of catalytic activity, and dysregulates the metabolic pathways [28, 29]. The protein oxidation is initiated by the abstraction of hydrogen from the protein by the hydroxyl radical and generates the

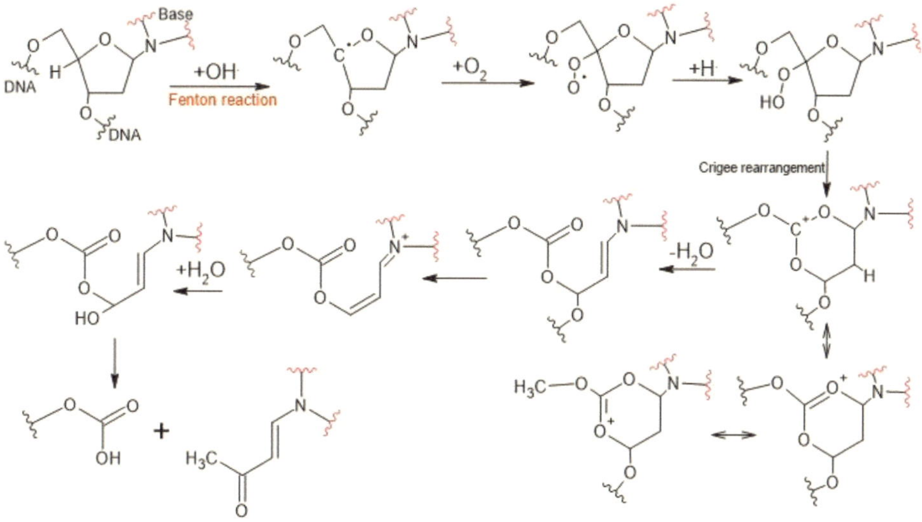

Figure 6.
Mechanism of oxidative damage to DNA-deoxyribose by Fenton and Haber-Weiss reaction [28].

protein radicals. It is stabilized by the resonance with the carboxyl group of protein. Then this protein radical reacts with oxygen and forms the protein peroxyl radical.

4. Conclusion

In summary, we described the regulatory mechanism of ROS production (mainly hydroxyl radicals) by Fenton and Haber-Weiss reaction. Created hydroxyl radicals facilitate ferroptosis, lipid peroxidation, DNA damage, and protein oxidation leading to epileptic episodes. Increasing evidence demonstrated that epilepsy is closely related to ferroptosis and iron metabolism. Ferroptosis is also accelerated by hydroxyl radical, which is mainly formed by Fenton and Haber-Weiss reaction. Therefore, antioxidant therapy, free radical scavenger therapy, and metal chelator therapy may be novel approaches to slow the progression of epilepsy. However, further investigation is needed for understanding new treatment strategies based on Fenton and Haber-Weiss's reaction to neurological diseases such as epilepsy.

Author details

Kaneez Fatima Shad[1,2,3*] and Tushar Kanti Das[4]

1 Ingham Institute for Applied Medical Research, Liverpool, NSW, Australia

2 School of Life Sciences, University of Technology Sydney, NSW, Australia

3 Faculty of Health Sciences, School of Behavioral and Health Sciences, Australian Catholic University, NSW, Australia

4 Department of Neurology, McGovern Medical School at the University of Texas Health Science Center at Houston, Houston, TX, USA

*Address all correspondence to: kaneez.Fatima-Shad@uts.edu.au; ftmshad@gmail.com

References

[1] Lee KH, Cha M, Lee BH. Neuroprotective effect of antioxidants in the brain. International Journal of Molecular Sciences. 2020;**21**(19):7152

[2] Aguiar CC, Almeida AB, Araújo PV, de Abreu RN, Chaves EM, do Vale OC, et al. Oxidative stress and epilepsy: Literature review. Oxidative Medicine and Cellular Longevity. 2012;**2012**: 795259

[3] Borowicz-Reutt KK, Czuczwar SJ. Role of oxidative stress in epileptogenesis and potential implications for therapy. Pharmacological Reports. 2020;**72**(5): 1218-1226

[4] Puttachary S, Sharma S, Stark S, Thippeswamy T. Seizure-induced oxidative stress in temporal lobe epilepsy. BioMed Research International. 2015;**2015**:745613

[5] Chen S, Chen Y, Zhang Y, Kuang X, Liu Y, Guo M, et al. Iron metabolism and Ferroptosis in epilepsy. Frontiers in Neuroscience. 2020;**14**:601193

[6] Fenton HJH. Oxidation of tartaric acid in presence of iron. Journal of the Chemical Society, Transactions. 1894;**65**: 899-910

[7] Ovalle R. A history of the Fenton reactions (Fenton chemistry for beginners). In: Reactive Oxygen Species. London, United Kingdom: IntechOpen Limited; 2022

[8] Barbusinski K. Fenton reaction-controversy concerning the chemistry. Ecological Chemistry and Engineering. 2009;**16**:347-358

[9] Kremer ML. New kinetic analysis of the Fenton reaction: Critical examination of the free radical – Chain reaction concept. Progress in Reaction Kinetics and Mechanism. 2019;**44**(4):289-299

[10] Ruben VM, Dorian PG, Michel V. Chapter 4 - Ferrioxalate-mediated processes. In: Ameta SC, Ameta R, editors. Advanced Oxidation Processes for Waste Water Treatment. Amsterdam, The Netherlands: Academic Press; 2018. pp. 89-113

[11] Pignatello JJ, Oliveros E, MacKay A. Advanced oxidation process for organic contaminant destruction based on the Fenton reaction. Critical Reviews in Environmental Science and Technology. 2006;**36**:1-84

[12] Paulina P, Filip M, Dawid Z, Kinga M. Agnieszka B decomposition of hydrogen perodixe - kinetics and review of chosen catalysts. Acta Innovations. 2018;**26**:45-52

[13] Rivas FJ, Beltran FJ, Frades J, Buxeda P. Oxidation of p-hydroxybenzoic acid by Fenton's reagent. Water Research. 2001;**35**:387-396

[14] Das TK, Wati MR, Shad KF. Oxidative stress gated by Fenton and Haber Weiss reactions and its association with Alzheimer's disease. Archives of Neuroscience. 2014;**2**(3):1-8

[15] Cai Y, Yang Z. Ferroptosis and its role in epilepsy. Frontiers in Cellular Neuroscience. 2021;**15**:1-10

[16] Geronzi U, Lotti F, Grosso S. Oxidative stress in epilepsy. Expert Review of Neurotherapeutics. 2018; **18**(5):427-434

[17] Dixon SJ, Lemberg KM, Lamprecht MR, Skouta R, Zaitsev EM,

Gleason CE, et al. Ferroptosis: An iron-dependent form of nonapoptotic cell death. Cell. 2012;**149**(5):1060-1072

[18] Zhao Y, Li X, Zhang K, Tong T, Cui R. The Progress of epilepsy after stroke. Current Neuropharmacology. 2018;**16**(1):71-78

[19] Myint PK, Staufenberg EF, Sabanathan K. Post-stroke seizure and post-stroke epilepsy. Postgraduate Medical Journal. 2006;**82**(971):568-572

[20] Wang Y, Wei P, Yan F, Luo Y, Zhao G. Animal models of epilepsy: A phenotype-oriented review. Aging and Disease. 2022;**13**(1):215-231

[21] Kundap UP, Paudel YN, Shaikh MF. Animal models of metabolic epilepsy and epilepsy associated metabolic dysfunction: A systematic review. Pharmaceuticals (Basel). 2020;**13**(6):106

[22] Zou X, Jiang S, Wu Z, Shi Y, Cai S, Zhu R, et al. Effectiveness of deferox-amine on ferric chloride-induced epilepsy in rats. Brain Research. 2017;**1658**:25-30

[23] Zimmer TS, David B, Broekaart DWM, et al. Seizure-mediated iron accumulation and dysregulated iron metabolism after status epilepticus and in temporal lobe epilepsy. Acta Neuropathologica. 2021;**142**:729-759

[24] Akyuz E, Doganyigit Z, Eroglu E, Moscovicz F, Merelli A, Lazarowski A, et al. Myocardial iron overload in an experimental model of sudden unexpected death in epilepsy. Frontiers in Neurology. 2021;**2021**(12):609236

[25] Andrews NC, Schmidt PJ. Iron homeostasis. Annual Review of Physiology. 2007;**69**:69-85

[26] Galaris D, Barbouti A, Pantopoulos K. Iron homeostasis and oxidative stress: An intimate relationship. Biochimica et Biophysica Acta Molecular Cell Research. 2019; **1866**:118535

[27] Dixon SJ, Winter GE, Musavi LS, Lee ED, Snijder B, Rebsamen M, et al. Human haploid cell genetics reveals roles for lipid metabolism genes in nonapoptotic cell death. ACS Chemical Biology. 2015;**2015**(10):1604-1609

[28] Juan CA, Pérez de la Lastra JM, Plou FJ, Pérez-Lebeña E. The chemistry of reactive oxygen species (ROS) revisited: Outlining their role in biological macromolecules (DNA, lipids and proteins) and induced pathologies. International Journal of Molecular Sciences. 2021;**22**(9):4642

[29] Iakovou E, Kourti M. A comprehensive overview of the complex role of oxidative stress in aging, the contributing environmental stressors and emerging antioxidant therapeutic interventions. Frontiers in Aging Neuroscience. 2022;**14**:827900

Chapter 2

The Role of Microglia in Neuroinflammation

Shao-Wen Hung, Chia-Chi Chen, Hsiao-Yun Chen, Ying-Ching Hung, Ping-Min Huang and Chia-Yu Lin

Abstract

Microglia typically exist in a resting state of a mature brain and monitors the brain environment. In response to brain injuries or immunological stimuli, however, microglia are readily activated. In their activated state, they can serve diverse beneficial functions essential for enhancing neuron survival through the release of trophic and anti-inflammatory factors. Under certain circumstances, such as sustained epilepsy, however, microglia become overactivated and can induce significant and highly detrimental neurotoxic effects by the excessive production of a large array of cytotoxic factors, such as nitric oxide and proinflammatory cytokines. Neuroinflammation has been identified in epileptogenic tissue and is suspected of participating in epileptogenesis. Recent evidence has shown the effects of anti-inflammation and protection against ischemic brain injury by inhibiting soluble epoxide hydrolase (sEH) pharmacologically and genetically. We assume that sEH inhibition might be also beneficial to prevent inflammatory processes caused by seizures and subsequent chronic epilepsy. In the present study, we investigated whether sEH is involved in overactivated microglia-induced neuroinflammation and subsequent epileptogenesis in a mouse model of temporal lobe epilepsy. Overactivated microglia will be detected by using imaging techniques. It is hoped that the results of the present study would provide a better understanding of the roles of sEH and microglia in epileptogenesis.

Keywords: epilepsy, epileptogenesis, microglia, neuroinflammation, soluble epoxide hydrolase

1. Introduction

Neuroinflammation has been identified in epilepsy-related tissue from both experimental and clinical evidence and is suspected to participate in the formation of neuronal cell death, reactive gliosis, and neuroplastic changes in the hippocampus, which may contribute to epileptogenesis [1–4]. The role of active microglia in neuroinflammation is tightly regulated under neurodegenerative processes. Therefore, the microglial regulation of neuroinflammation may provide a therapeutic target for the treatment of severe or chronic neuroinflammation (**Figure 1**).

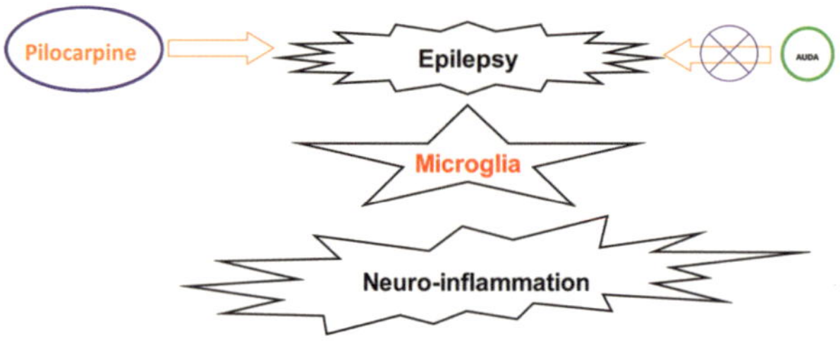

Figure 1.
The relationship of neuroinflammation and epileptogenesis. Pilocarpine induces epilepsy. AUDA suppress epilepsy. Microglia plays an important role between epilepsy and neuroinflammation.

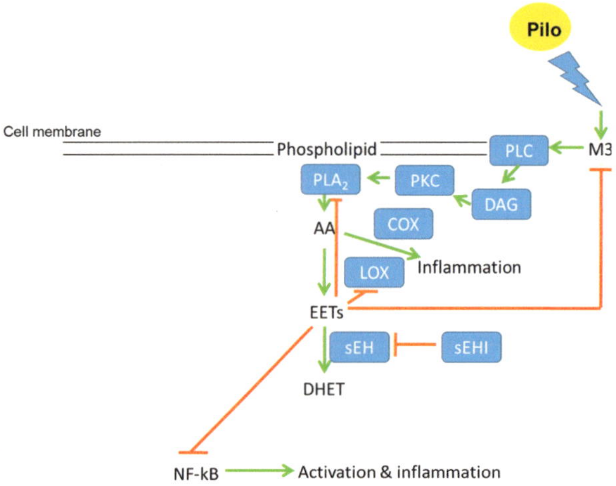

Figure 2.
The mechanism of pilocarpine (pilo) and sEH in the activation and inflammation in microglia. Muscarinic acetylcholine receptor (M3), PLC (phospholipase C), PLA_2 (phospholipases A_2), PKC (protein kinase C), DAG (diacylglycerol), COX (cyclooxygenase), LOX (lipoxygenase), sEH (soluble epoxide hydrolase), sEHI (soluble epoxide hydrolase inhibitors), AA (arachidonic acid), EETs (epoxyeicosatrienoic acids), DHET (dihydroxyeicosatrienoic acids), and NF-kB (nuclear factor kappa-light-chain-enhancer of activated B cells) play in the neuroinflammation. Pilo causes the neuroinflammation and epileptogenesis. 12-(3-Adamantan-1-yl-ureido)-dodecanoic acid (AUDA) suppress epilepsy.

During neuroinflammation, the pro-inflammatory-related cytokines, such as tumor necrosis factor-alpha (TNF-α), interleukin-6 (IL-6), and interleukin-1β (IL-1β), are produced by active microglia or astrocytes and next provoked pathological signaling cascades through phospholipase C and phospholipase A2 activations [5, 6]. Finally, the oxidized enzymes released the non-esterified arachidonic acid (AA) from cellular phospholipids and the formation of lysophospholipids and bioactive eicosanoids (**Figure 2**).

2. Epilepsy and treatments in people

In total, 1–3% of people in the world approximately suffer from epilepsy. Pharmacotherapy is the main treatment for most epileptic patients [7–10]. Moreover, the surgery is another option for epileptic patients according to the clinical doctors' diagnosis by referring to brain imaging and seizure mapping techniques. When epileptic patients cannot control seizures, by treatment with antiepileptic drugs (AEDs) or are not viable for surgery, vagal nerve stimulation will be a third possible option [11–16]. Unfortunately, a number of epileptic patients cannot control seizures. Herein, it is needed to research and develop more efficacious therapies for these epileptic patients with uncontrolled seizures [17–20].

3. The role of enzyme systems in the neuroinflammation

The cyclooxygenases, lipoxygenases, and cytochrome P450 (CYP) epoxygenases participated in metabolizing released AA to lipid metabolites as leukotrienes, epoxyeicosatrienoic acids (EETs), and prostaglandins (**Figure 2**). Brain parenchymal tissue metabolizes AA to EETs via the CYP epoxygenase, which regulates cerebral blood flow (CBF) and against neuroinflammation and apoptosis. Recently, hypoxia and ischemic preconditioning experiments have shown that the increased expression of CYP epoxygenase and EETs in the brain may confer protection from an ischemic stroke induced by middle cerebral artery occlusion (MCAO) in the animal model. It also suggests that EETs signaling may suppress the ischemia-evoked inflammatory cytokine response in the brain, supporting an anti-neuroinflammatory role for EETs in the brain circulation [21–28].

Iba1 is specifically expressed in microglia or macrophages and is up-regulated during the activation of these cells following nerve injury, central nervous system ischemia, and several other brain diseases. Additionally, whether soluble epoxide hydrolase (sEH) expression in the microglia should be verified? sEH can perform the metabolic conversion of EETs into their less active form as dihydroxyeicosatrienoic acids. Currently, the inhibition of sEH has been used to increase systemic EETs level and bioactivity. Through applying the pharmacologic inhibitors or genetic deletion, the inhibition of sEH attenuated the cerebral ischemia-induced vascular and neural injury, suggesting sEH might be a novel target for stroke treatment [29–37].

4. Experimental design *in vitro* for evaluating the role of microglia in Neuroinflammation

The reagents were ordered and prepared to perform *in vitro* experiment. The 12-(3-Adamantan-1-yl-ureido)-dodecanoic acid (AUDA) was ordered from Cayman Chemical (Ann Arbor, MI, USA) and dissolved in dimethyl sulfoxide (DMSO; Cat No. 472301; Sigma-Aldrich, MO, USA). Pilocarpine was ordered and dissolved in 0.9% saline. The 90% ethanol (Sigma-Aldrich), Liu's stain (ASK, Taoyuan, and Taiwan), and Griess reagent system (Promega, Madison, and WI) were ordered. Cytofix/Cytoperm™ (BD Biosciences, CA, USA), Perm/Wash™ (BD Biosciences), mouse anti- Iba1 monoclonal antibody (sc-52,328; Santa Cruz Biotechnology), mouse anti-sEH monoclonal antibody (sc-6260; Santa Cruz Biotechnology), and FITC-labeled goat anti-mouse IgG antibody (1:1000) (sc-2010; Santa Cruz Biotechnology) were ordered for the determination of activated microglial marker and sEH expression by flow cytometric assay. The 3-(4,5-Dimethyl- 2-thiazolyl)-2,5-diphenyl-2H-tetrazolium bromide (MTT, MERCK, Darmstadt, Germany) was ordered and dissolved in 1× phosphate-buffered saline (PBS; Sigma-Aldrich).

Mouse retroviral immortalized microglia BV-2 cells belonging to the C57BL/6 background were grown in Dulbecco's modified Eagle's medium (DMEM) supplemented with 10% fetal bovine serum (FBS; Gibco®), 2 mM L-glutamine, 100 U/mL penicillin (Sigma-Aldrich), and 100 μg/mL streptomycin (Sigma-Aldrich) in 5% CO_2 atmosphere at 37°C. Cells were treated with 100 μM pilocarpine and/or 100 μM AUDA and cultured for 24 hrs in 10% FBS-DMEM on glass coverslips. Observation of cell morphology with/without treatment was done by light microscope (Olympus CKX41, Olympus Optical Co. Ltd.). Cells were grown to 90% confluency before the experiments.

Measurement of cell viability was measured by MTT assay according to the manufacturer's instructions. At the experimental points, cell viability was detected by MTT assay. The reduced purple dye intensity of color was estimated by reading at an optical density of 570 nm in a spectrophotometer. Moreover, *In vitro* migration assays (scratch assay and transwell migration assay) were performed. Scratch assays were performed following the previously described. Briefly, the BV-2 microglia in six well plates were performed with serum-free DMEM for three wash times. A line down the center of each well was scraped with a sterile p200 pipette tip and followed by a wash step to remove debris with serum-free DMEM. Images were taken at 10× magnification of the light microscopy (Olympus BX43, Olympus Optical Co. Ltd.). The scratch widths were measured and wound closure was calculated by dividing widths measured after 8 hours of incubation by the initial scraped width. Each experiment was carried out in triplicate and three fields were blindly counted per well by scorers. Transwell migration assays were performed by using Boyden chambers (BD Bioscience). The 4×10^4 BV-2 microglia (200 μL serum-free DMEM) were added to the upper chamber of Boyden chambers and allowed to adhere to the polycarbonate filters (8 μm pore) for 30 mins at 37°C in a humidified atmosphere of 95% air and 5% CO_2. Following this, BV-2 microglia were treated with 100 μM pilocarpine at 37°C for 30 mins prior to AUDA treatment. The 100 μM AUDA was then placed in the upper chamber and the lower chamber was added with 10% fetal bovine serum (FBS)-DMEM to attract BV-2 microglia migration. BV-2 cells did not migrate and remained on the upper surface of the Boyden chambers' filter were removed. BV-2 cells that had migrated to the lower surface were fixed with 90% ethanol, stained with Liu's stain (ASK, Taoyuan, Taiwan), and counted. In at least three independent experiments, three wells per treatment were blindly counted in nine random fields at 40× magnification per well by scorers.

A phagocytosis assay was performed in this experiment. BV-2 microglia seeded in six well plates were incubated with 100 μM pilocarpine at 37°C for 30 mins prior to 100 μM AUDA treatment for 24 hrs. After 24 hrs treatment, the phagocytic ability of the microglia was measured by using FITC-labeled dextran (MW 40,000) as a tracer. Briefly, microglia were exposed to 30 μg/mL FITC-labeled dextran for 30 mins. Later, three washing times with cold PBS (pH 7.4) were performed prior to measuring fluorescence at 480 nm excitation and 520 nm emission on a flow cytometer (FACS Calibular, BD Biosciences) or fluorescence microscopy (Olympus BX43, Olympus Optical). As a background, the cultures without FITC-dextran were used. Each culture condition was performed in quadruplicate, and three independent experiments were performed.

Measurement of extracellular nitric oxide production was performed. The nitrite, a stable breakdown product of nitric oxide, was measured with a Griess Reagent System (Promega, Madison, WI). Determination of activated microglial marker and sEH expression by flow cytometric assay was performed. First, BV-2 cells were pretreated with 100 μM pilocarpine for 30 mins then were treated with 100 μM AUDA for 24 hrs in 10% FBS with DMEM. After pilocarpine-AUDA co-treatment, these cells were harvested and fixed in Cytofix/Cytoperm™ (BD Biosciences) at 4°C for 15 mins and washed twice with 1× Perm/Wash™ (BD Biosciences). Fixed cells were stained with various primary antibodies [mouse anti-Iba1 monoclonal antibody (1:100

dilution) (sc-52,328; Santa Cruz Biotechnology) and mouse anti-sEH monoclonal antibody (1:100 dilution) (sc-6260; Santa Cruz Biotechnology)] at 4°C for 30 mins and then washed twice with 1× Perm/Wash™ (BD Biosciences). Secondary antibodies [FITC-labeled goat anti-mouse IgG antibody (1:1000 dilution) (sc-2010; Santa Cruz Biotechnology)] were subsequently stained at 4°C for 30 mins. Finally, cells were stained with 5 μg/mL PI (propidium iodide; BD Biosciences) at room temperature for 5 mins. Cells were analyzed by a flow cytometer (FACSCalibur, BD Biosciences) and WinMDI software (version 2.9). Statistical analysis was performed in this study. The values are reported as mean ± SE. All statistical comparisons were made with two-tailed tests. Statistical evaluation was performed using Student's *t*-test, one-way ANOVA, and/or Dunnett's post hoc test. Differences between groups were considered statistically significant at $^{**}p < 0.01$ and $^{***}p < 0.001$.

5. AUDA significantly inhibited pilocarpine-induce BV-2 microglial activation and cytokine expressions

The 100 μM pilocarpine did not affect cell viability and the half-maximal inhibitory concentration (IC_{50}) was 17.5 mM. The 100 μM AUDA did not affect cell viability and the

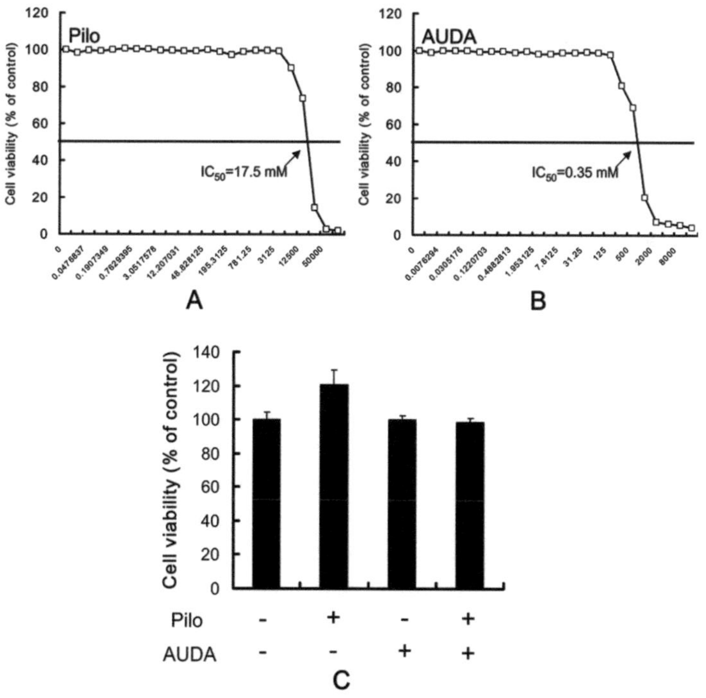

Figure 3.
BV-2 microglial cell viability for the pilocarpine and/or AUDA treatment. (A) BV-2 cells treated with the serial two-fold diluted concentration of pilocarpine (0 to 100,000 μM) at 37°C for 24 hrs in 10% serum-DMEM. Cell viability was determined by using MTT assay. The half maximal inhibitory concentration (IC_{50}) of pilocarpine was 17.5 mM. (B) BV-2 cells treated with the serial two-fold diluted concentration of AUDA (0 to 16,000 μM) at 37°C for 24 hrs in 10% serum-DMEM. Cell viability was determined by using MTT assay. 100 μM pilocarpine did not affect cell viability and the half maximal inhibitory concentration (IC_{50}) of AUDA was 0.35 mM. (C) Non-cytotoxic concentration (100 μM) of pilocarpine and AUDA were used in this study. Non-cytotoxic effect was presented after 100 μM pilocarpine combined with 100 μM AUDA treatment at 37°C for 24 hrs in 10% serum-DMEM. Values are reported as mean ± SE.

half-maximal inhibitory concentration (IC_{50}) was 0.35 mM. Non-cytotoxic concentration (100 μM) of pilocarpine and AUDA were used in this study (**Figure 3A** and **B**). The non-cytotoxic effect was presented after 100 μM pilocarpine combined with 100 μM AUDA treatment (**Figure 3C**). The mean fluorescence intensity (MFI) of Iba1 expression was significantly increased in the BV-2 microglial cells under direct 100 μM pilocarpine

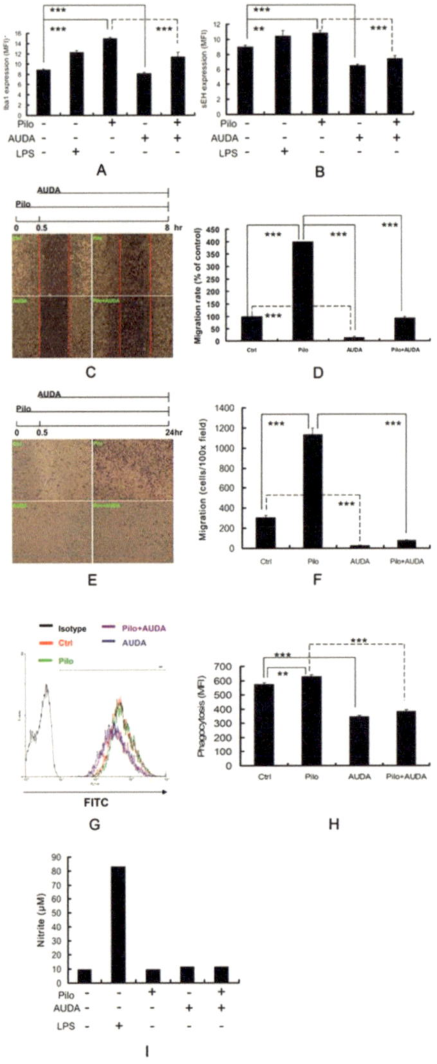

Figure 4.

AUDA significantly inhibited pilocarpine-induce BV-2 microglial activation and cytokine expressions. (A) MFI of Iba1 expression was significantly increased in the BV-2 microglial cells under the direct 100 μM pilocarpine stimulation. AUDA significantly decreased Iba1 expression. (B) sEH expression was presented in the BV-2 microglia. 100 μM AUDA significantly decreased sEH expression in BV-2 microglia. (C, D) AUDA significantly suppressed pilocarpine-active BV-2 cell migration by using wound-healing assay. (E, F) AUDA significantly suppressed pilocarpine-active BV-2 cell migration by using Boyden chamber assay. (G, H) histogram showed 100% phagocytosis in all groups. AUDA significantly suppressed phagocytic abilities of pilocarpine-active BV-2 cells by using flow cytometry. (I) No effects of nitric oxide production were presented in all groups. Values are reported as mean ± SE. All statistical comparisons were made with two-tailed tests. Statistical evaluation was performed using Student's t-test. Differences between groups were considered statistically significant at $^{**}p < 0.01$; $^{***}p < 0.001$.

stimulation (**Figure 4A**). The sEH expression was presented in the BV-2 microglia (**Figure 4B**). C-terminal inhibitor of she, AUDA (100 μM), significantly decreased Iba1 and sEH expressions in the active BV2 microglia (**Figure 4A** and **B**). After microglial activation, cell migration, phagocytosis, and cytotoxicity were enhanced. According to these results, AUDA significantly suppressed cell migration, and phagocytosis (**Figure 4C–H**). Additionally, alone or combined pilocarpine or AUDA treatment did not affect extracellular nitric oxide production in BV-2 microglia (**Figure 4I**).

6. Discussion

Epilepsy affects approximately 1–3% population of the world, and temporal lobe epilepsy (TLE) is the most common localized epilepsy disorder, accounting for approximately 40% of adults with epilepsy [38]. However, the exact mechanism for the formation of TLE remains unclear. According to the engulfment-promoted cell death theory, nerve cells have special receptors. When nerve cells are injured, activated microglia will recognize this receptor and contact nerve cells, indirectly causing nerve cell death [39]. In addition, some studies have confirmed that microglia can also be directly activated by some activating factors, thereby affecting the function and survival of nerve cells [39]. Previous studies have confirmed that the EETs-sEH pathway is associated with brain inflammation, but whether the EETs-sEH pathway is involved in the formation of TLE remains to be clarified. For these reasons, studying the molecular and cellular mechanisms of the brain's transition from normal to epilepsy can be used to understand the neurobiological changes in epilepsy formation and provide a new therapeutic strategy. Therefore, this study hopes to find a new treatment by understanding the performance and function of sEH microglia in the resting state and the microglia in the activated state, and using the functional inhibitor of sEH to find out how to regulate the activation of microglia. The method of epilepsy is expected to provide clinicians with a reference for the treatment of epilepsy and the use of AEDs in the future. This study demonstrated that AUDA, an inhibitor of sEH, significantly inhibited sEH expression and pilocarpine-induced microglia activation, including phagocytosis and migration. From these results, pilocarpine can directly activate microglia, and inhibition of the EET-sEH pathway can inhibit activated microglia, including phagocytosis and migration. Based on these research results, it is hoped that in the future, it will be helpful to neuroscience researchers in molecular and cellular research on the pathogenic mechanism of TLE, and provide clinicians with a reference for treating epilepsy and the use of anti-epileptic drugs.

7. Conclusions

Neurological disorders are complicated in the brain and spinal cord and are caused by a loss of neurons and glial cells in these injured areas. Currently, neurological disorders can affect hundreds of millions of people worldwide. More than 50 million people have epilepsy worldwide. The microglia are a key causative factor in the process of neuroinflammation. Commonly, microglia are activated after the brain injury and the activated microglia can induce neurocytotoxic factors. At present, much evidence have demonstrated microglial activation following pilocarpine-induced seizures. Our results suggest a role for sEH in regulating epileptogenesis of

BV-2 microglia *in vitro*, whereas the effect of hydrolase inhibition on epileptogenesis may provide a novel therapeutic approach for approximately 20–40% of the clinically anti-epileptic drugs-uncontrolled epileptic patients.

Acknowledgements

The authors thank the Ministry of Science and Technology and the Council of Agriculture, Taiwan for support. The plan number of Council of Agriculture is 111AS-11.3.2-ST-a2.

Conflict of interest

The authors declare no conflict of interest.

Author details

Shao-Wen Hung*, Chia-Chi Chen, Hsiao-Yun Chen, Ying-Ching Hung, Ping-Min Huang and Chia-Yu Lin
Division of Animal Industry, Animal Technology Research Center, Agricultural Technology Research Institute, Hsinchu, Taiwan

*Address all correspondence to: 1032169@mail.atri.org.tw

References

[1] Hung YW, Lai MT, Tseng YJ, Chou CC, Lin YY. Monocyte chemoattractant protein-1 affects migration of hippocampal neural progenitors following status epilepticus in rats. Journal of Neuroinflammation. 2013;**10**:11

[2] Hung YW, Yang DI, Huang PY, Lee TS, Kuo TBJ, Yiu CH, et al. The duration of sustained convulsive seizures determines the pattern of hippocampal neurogenesis and the development of spontaneous epilepsy in rats. Epilepsy Research. 2012;**98**:206-215

[3] DeLorenzo RJ, Hauser WA, Towne AR, Boggs JG, Pellock JM, Penberthy L, et al. A prospective, population-based epidemiologic study of status epilepticus in Richmond, Virginia. Neurology. 1996;**46**:1029-1035

[4] Hanna J, Nichol A. Status epilepticus: an intensive care medicine problem. Anaesthesia & Intensive Care Medicine. 2012;**13**:148-151

[5] Marchi N, Oby E, Batra A, Uva L, De Curtis M, Hernandez N, et al. *In vivo* and *in vitro* effects of pilocarpine: Relevance to ictogenesis. Epilepsia. 2007;**48**:1934-1946

[6] Wang CH, Hung CP, Chen MT, Shih YH, Lin YY. Hippocampal desynchronization of functional connectivity prior to the onset of status epilepticus in pilocarpine-treated rats. PLoS One. 2012;7:e39763

[7] Vissers C, Ming GL, Song H. Nanoparticle technology and stem cell therapy team up against neurodegenerative disorders. Advanced Drug Delivery Reviews. 2019;**148**:239-251

[8] Loscher W. Molecular mechanisms of drug resistance in status epilepticus. Epilepsia. 2009;**50**(Suppl. 12):19-21

[9] Alldredge BK, Gelb AM, Isaacs SM, Corry MD, Allen F, Ulrich S, et al. A comparison of lorazepam, diazepam, and placebo for the treatment of out-of-hospital status epilepticus. New England Journal of Medicine. 2001;**345**:631-637

[10] Alvarez V, Januel JM, Burnand B, Rossetti AO. Second-line status epilepticus treatment: Comparison of phenytoin, valproate, and levetiracetam. Epilepsia. 2011;**52**:1292-1296

[11] Claassen J, Hirsch LJ, Emerson RG, Mayer SA. Treatment of refractory status epilepticus with pentobarbital, propofol, or midazolam: A systematic review. Epilepsia. 2002;**43**:146-153

[12] French JA. Response to early AED therapy and its prognostic implications. Epilepsy Currents. 2002;**2**:69-71

[13] Wahab A, Albus K, Gabriel S, Heinemann U. In search of models of pharmacoresistant epilepsy. Epilepsia. 2010;**51**(Suppl. 3):154-159

[14] Song CG, Zhang YZ, Wu HN, Cao XL, Guo CJ, Li YQ, et al. Stem cells: A promising candidate to treat neurological disorders. Neural Regeneration Research. 2018;**13**:1294-1304

[15] Ravizza T, Gagliardi B, Noe F, Boer K, Aronica E, Vezzani A. Innate and adaptive immunity during epileptogenesis and spontaneous seizures: Evidence from experimental models and human temporal lobe epilepsy. Neurobiology of Disease. 2008;**29**:142-160

[16] Vezzani A, Granata T. Brain inflammation in epilepsy: Experimental and clinical evidence. Epilepsia. 2005;**46**:1724-1743

[17] Jakubs K, Bonde S, Iosif RE, Ekdahl CT, Kokaia Z, Kokaia M, et al. Inflammation regulates functional integration of neurons born in adult brain. Journal of Neuroscience. 2008;**28**:12477-12488

[18] Choi J, Koh S. Role of brain inflammation in epileptogenesis. Yonsei Medical Journal. 2008;**49**:1-18

[19] Turrin NP, Rivest S. Innate immune reaction in response to seizures: Implications for the neuropathology associated with epilepsy. Neurobiology of Disease. 2004;**16**:321-334

[20] Vezzani A, French J, Bartfai T, Baram TZ. The role of inflammation in epilepsy. Nature Reviews Neurology. 2011;**7**:31-40

[21] Fritschy JM. Epilepsy, E/I balance and GABA(a) receptor plasticity. Frontiers Research Foundation. 2008;**1**:5

[22] Scharfman HE, Smith KL, Goodman JH, Sollas AL. Survival of dentate hilar mossy cells after pilocarpine-induced seizures and their synchronized burst discharges with area CA3 pyramidal cells. Neuroscience. 2001;**104**:741-759

[23] Isokawa M. Decrement of GABAA receptor-mediated inhibitory postsynaptic currents in dentate granule cells in epileptic hippocampus. Journal of Neurophysiology. 1996;**75**:1901-1908

[24] Wiebe SP, Staubli UV. Recognition memory correlates of hippocampal theta cells. Journal of Neuroscience. 2001;**21**:3955-3967

[25] Williams PA, Wuarin JP, Dou P, Ferraro DJ, Dudek FE. Reassessment of the effects of cycloheximide on mossy fiber sprouting and epileptogenesis in the pilocarpine model of temporal lobe epilepsy. Journal of Neurophysiology. 2002;**88**:2075-2087

[26] Hung YW, Hung SW, Wu YC, Wong LK, Lai MT, Shih YH, et al. Soluble epoxide hydrolase activity regulates inflammatory responses and seizure generation in two mouse models of temporal lobe epilepsy. Brain Behavior and Immunity. 2015;**43**:118-129

[27] Vezzani A, Moneta D, Richichi C, Aliprandi M, Burrows SJ, Ravizza T, et al. Functional role of inflammatory cytokines and antiinflammatory molecules in seizures and epileptogenesis. Epilepsia. 2002;**43**(Suppl. 5):30-35

[28] Hopkins SJ, Rothwell NJ. Cytokines and the nervous system. I: Expression and recognition. Trends in Neurosciences. 1995;**18**:83-88

[29] Aisen PS, Davis KL. Inflammatory mechanisms in Alzheimer's disease: Implications for therapy. American Journal of Psychiatry. 1994;**151**:1105-1113

[30] Hauss-Wegrzyniak B, Dobrzanski P, Stoehr JD, Wenk GL. Chronic neuroinflammation in rats reproduces components of the neurobiology of Alzheimer's disease. Brain Research. 1998;**780**:294-303

[31] Lee SC, Han JS, Seo JK, Cha YN. Modulation of cyclooxygenase-2 expression by phosphatidylcholine specific phospholipase C and D in macrophages stimulated with lipopolysaccharide. Molecules and Cells. 2003;**15**:320-326

[32] Balsinde J, Winstead MV, Dennis EA. Phospholipase a(2)

regulation of arachidonic acid mobilization. FEBS Letters. 2002;**531**:2-6

[33] Rosenberger TA, Villacreses NE, Hovda JT, Bosetti F, Weerasinghe G, Wine RN, et al. Rat brain arachidonic acid metabolism is increased by a 6-day intracerebral ventricular infusion of bacterial lipopolysaccharide. Journal of Neurochemistry. 2004;**88**:1168-1178

[34] Shimizu T, Wolfe LS. Arachidonic acid cascade and signal transduction. Journal of Neurochemistry. 1990;**55**:1-15

[35] Crespel A, Coubes P, Rousset MC, Brana C, Rougier A, Rondouin G, et al. Inflammatory reactions in human medial temporal lobe epilepsy with hippocampal sclerosis. Brain Research. 2002;**952**:159-169

[36] Jankowsky JL, Patterson PH. The role of cytokines and growth factors in seizures and their sequelae. Progress in Neurobiology. 2001;**63**:125-149

[37] Vezzani A, Balosso S, Ravizza T. The role of cytokines in the pathophysiology of epilepsy. Brain, Behavior, and Immunity. 2008;**22**:797-803

[38] Loo LS, McNamara JO. Impaired volume regulation is the mechanism of excitotoxic sensitization to complement. Journal of Biomedical Science. 2006;**26**:10177-10187

[39] Marín-Teva JL, Dusart I, Colin C, Gervais A, Rooijen NV, Mallat M. Microglia promote the death of developing Purkinje cells. Neuron. 2004;**41**:535-547

Chapter 3

Epileptic Focus in Drug-Resistant Epilepsy: Structure, Organization, and Pathophysiology

Yulia M. Zabrodskaya, Olga N. Gaykova, Mikhail V. Alexandrov, Natalia M. Paramonova, Darya A. Sitovskaya, Anastasya V. Litovchenko, Tatiana V. Sokolova, Sofiia E. Cherenkova and Elena D. Bazhanova

Abstract

The chapter focuses on how different cutting-edge techniques can be used to study electrophysiological, pathomorphological, and biochemical changes in the "epileptic focus" area of the cerebral cortex and white matter to see how epileptic seizures become drug-resistant and how it affects the other regions of the brain. The authors highlight the significance of neuroinflammation and apoptosis in the epilepsy pathogenesis providing EEG characteristics and describing structural changes in the cortex and white matter under such conditions as focal cortical dysplasia and epileptic leukoencephalopathy. Particular focus is given to structural and functional changes in the hippocampus and the role of hippocampal sclerosis in epilepsy. Key conceptions regarding the epileptic focus formation are outlined.

Keywords: drug-resistant epilepsy, epileptic focus, pathomorphology, FCD, hippocampal sclerosis, leukoencephalopathy, apoptosis, neuroinflammation

1. Introduction

The mechanisms leading to the development of epilepsy have become an area of active research. There is still no pathogenetic treatment for epilepsy, and there is no way to prevent this pathology development [1] with focal temporal lobe epilepsy being the most frequent type (approximately 80% of cases) [2]. The disease progression from the "epileptic neuron" to the "epileptic brain" and an increase in mental and cognitive disorders remain problems beyond solution for epileptology [1, 3–5]. Structural forms of epilepsy are the most difficult for drug correction, and most of them belong to drug-resistant epilepsy (DRE). Mesial temporal epilepsy, the structural basis of which is mesial temporal sclerosis, or hippocampal sclerosis is a more common form of temporal epilepsy. The etiopathogenesis of mesial temporal sclerosis has been the subject of active discussion since its first description by Sommer [6]. While the pathogenesis of hippocampal sclerosis remains a controversial and unclear issue, the role of the hippocampus in the development of medial temporal epilepsy is obvious. In the absence of effective medical treatment, the only effective, however the most radical, way is surgical intervention, in which the affected area of the brain is isolated and removed, which can help get rid of epileptic seizures. However, only half of the patients show positive results [3]. It is the heterogeneity of structural lesions and significant differences in functional and molecular biological state of cells that can play a key role not only in the pathogenesis of epilepsy but also in triggering insensitivity to drug therapy, as well as in determining the disease prognosis [7].

2. Neurophysiological correlates structural and functional disorders in temporal lobe epilepsy

2.1 Functional zones of the epileptic focus

The pathogenetic basis of epilepsy is the pathological system of the epileptic focus formed by constellations of neurons with grossly altered excitability parameters, which underpins their tendency to hypersynchronization and generation of discharge activity [8]. An epileptic focus displays the properties of a pathological determinant in the formation of a pathological system.

An epileptic focus should be considered as a set of several zones, each of which determines its own aspect in the clinical and neurophysiological picture of epilepsy: (1) the seizure-onset zone, (2) the symptomatogenic zone, (3) the zone of irritation (irritation), (4) the zone of functional deficiency, and (5) the zone of epileptogenic damage (epileptogenic focus) (**Figure 1**). The concept of focal epilepsy implies the presence of the so-called epileptogenic zone—a set of pathologically altered neuronal formations that make up the determinant generator in the epileptic system [8, 9]. Effective surgical treatment is believed to depend on the possibility to remove the epileptogenic zone, which results in complete release from seizures.

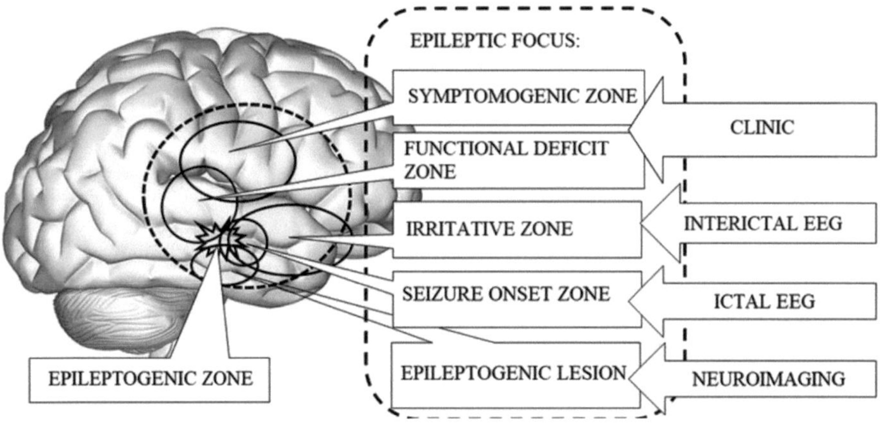

Figure 1.
Structural and functional organization of epileptic focus (scheme).

The zone of epileptogenic damage is an area of structural changes in brain tissues. Intrahemispheric and convexital tumors, cavernomas, arteriovenous malformations, and other structural changes may be associated with the development of epilepsy. These forms of epilepsy are qualified as structural epilepsy (in previous classifications—symptomatic epilepsy). Neuroimaging studies are conducted to identify epileptogenic damage.

The symptomatogenic zone is an area of the cortex, the activation of which during the circulation of epileptic discharges forms a clinical picture of a typical epileptic seizure for a patient. For greater accuracy of localization of the symptomatogenic zone, video recording of the seizure is used. Detailed clinical manifestations of the seizure are formed with a significant spread of pathological activity in the cortex. Consequently, the symptomatogenic zone is often more widespread than the seizure-onset zone. *The zone of functional deficiency* is an area of the cortex, the dysfunction of which in the post-access (less often—in the inter-access) period determines the clinical symptoms of "loss."

The seizure-onset area, that is, the cortex area generating hypersynchronous discharge activity when an epileptic attack occurs is the closest to the epileptogenic zone. To localize the seizure onset, an attack (ictal) should be registered with electroencephalography (EEG) and video recording of an ictal event. The irritative zone in the cortex is localized by the interstitial (interictal) epileptiform activity registered on the EEG [10].

2.2 Epileptic focus identification

To accurately localize the epileptic focus, for surgical resection purposes including, all patients undergo a comprehensive clinical neurological and electrophysiological examination (EEG), video EEG registering an epileptic seizure typical for a patient, in some cases invasive monitoring is carried out, neuroimaging examination (high-field magnetic resonance imaging (MRI) and positron emission tomography).

The reference method for detecting the zone of epileptic activity with structural temporal epilepsy is scalping video EEG monitoring when an ictal event is registered. In a complex diagnostic situation, when the scalping EEG does not allow to accurately localize the seizure-onset area, continuous invasive monitoring of the bioelectric activity of the brain is recommended [11]. When clinical and electroencephalographic data indicate possible involvement of the hippocampal complex in the epileptic system, invasive monitoring of the bioelectric activity of deep brain structures is performed: Spenser-type electrodes are installed stereotaxically in the basal and medial parts of the temporal cortex, in the hippocampus and amygdala, and less often in other structures. The choice of target structures is based on clinical picture analysis, scalp video EEG monitoring results, and ictal events semiology [12].

2.3 Bioelectric activity of the hippocampus

The dominance of slow-wave delta-band activity has been shown to be the distinctive feature of bioelectric activity tracks in the presence of hippocampal sclerosis as it accounts for up to 50% of the spectral power (**Figure 2**). Bioelectric activity tracks registered in the hippocampus without signs of structural lesions were not parametrically homogeneous. Two subgroups were clearly distinguished: a subgroup of hippocampus with bioelectric activity parameters similar to the group of damaged hippocampus and a subgroup of hippocampus, the spectral composition of activity of

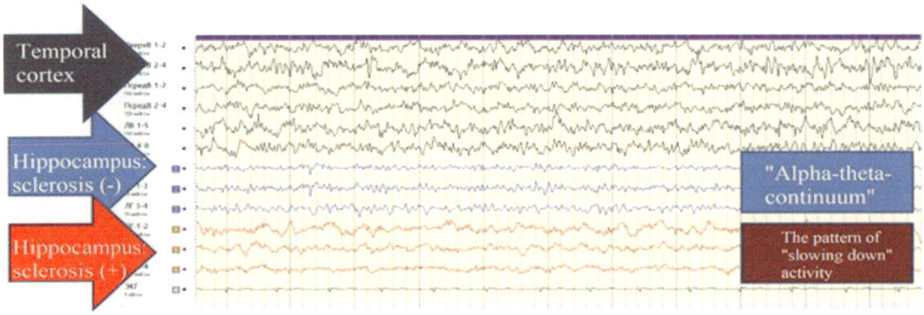

Figure 2.
Extraoperative monitoring of bioelectrical activity of the temporal cortex and hippocampus.

which was mainly in the alpha range. The similarity of the parameters of bioelectric activity in the second subgroup and in the group with obvious structural changes in the hippocampus suggests that hippocampal lesions did not reach the level necessary for damage signs neuroimaging, but the compromise of the hippocampus was sufficient to form a slow-wave pattern of "loss of activity" [13].

To clarify the mechanisms of bioelectric activity formation in the hippocampal complex, we performed a coherent analysis of amplitude-frequency parameters. Low coherence values in the analyzed lead pairs allow concluding that the bioelectric activity recorded in the hippocampus area is generated by the hippocampus itself and do not originate in the nearby areas of the temporal lobe cortex. Of course, it is not possible to completely exclude the possibility of electrical activity from brain areas in which invasive electrodes have not been implanted. However, this process is unlikely, judging by very low values of the coherence coefficients in the lead pairs under study.

Thus, bioelectric activity of the hippocampal complex in its structural lesion specifically features stable registration of the epileptiform activity of the average index with delta activity domineering and making up to 40–50% of the spectral power [13]. In the absence of neuroimaging signs of hippocampal complex structural lesions, the pattern of bioelectric activity can be predominantly formed by the activity of *theta* and *alpha* frequency ranges and may be similar to the slow-wave pattern in hippocampal sclerosis. This may be another evidence of the unified thalamic mechanisms of generating activity of alpha and theta frequency ranges known as the "alpha-theta continuum" conception [14, 15].

2.4 General anesthesia effects on the hippocampus bioelectric activity in epilepsy

When performing intraoperative examinations, it is important to take into account the general anesthesia type. Total intravenous anesthesia using drugs, such as propofol, which have a pronounced GABA-positive effect, in medium-effective doses causes the generation of high-frequency activity [16]. This makes it difficult to verify discharge epileptiform activity on electrocorticography (ECoG) and on electrosubcorticography (EsubCoG). In this regard, during neurosurgical operations, which are performed on patients with DRE, preference is given to inhaled anesthetics (**Figure 3**).

At the same time, the dose of a general anesthetic should not cause the formation of periodic flash-suppression patterns on the ECoG, and even more so on the EEG, since with such deep depression, epileptiform stigmata are either not registered [17, 18] or the source of their generation becomes difficult to localize [19, 20].

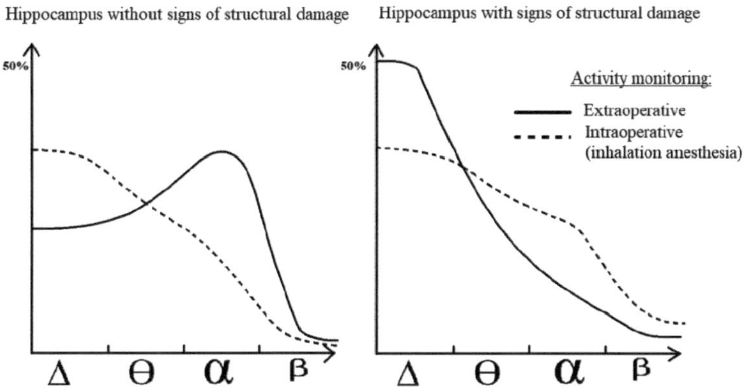

Figure 3.
Changes in the amplitude-frequency parameters of the bioelectrical activity of the hippocampal complexes under the action of inhalation anesthetic sevoflurane (scheme).

3. Pathomorphology of epileptic foci

3.1 Structural heterogeneity of the epileptic focus

Morphological studies of the brain in epilepsy have been actively conducted for 60–70 years. Structural changes in people suffering from epilepsy were found to be nonspecific and occur in different combinations in almost all patients. When studying the issues of epileptic foci localization, more attention is paid to the verification of nosologically determined forms of pathologies (tumor, malformations, etc.) and the so-called "sclerosis" of the hippocampus, which are attributed to the epileptogenic component of the epileptic system [21, 22]. Most studies of the epileptic activity zone focused on the neuronal complexes of the cortex and subcortical formations, and more specifically, on a damaged ("sick") neuron, or rather, a group of neurons capable of generating overexcitation with its spread to other brain structures or to the brain as a whole. However, epilepsy of different origins reveals significant structural changes not only in the gray but also in the white matter of the brain. However, little attention is paid to nonspecific morphofunctional characteristics of changes developing in the epileptic focus [22, 23].

During the pathomorphological examination of biopsies of the temporal lobe and hippocampus from the epileptic foci zone, a permanent complex of pathomorphological changes is verified, representing a combination of various pathological processes of both dysplastic and secondary degenerative-dystrophic and reactive-adaptive nature, accompanied by the development of substitutive gliosis and atrophy, including the hippocampal formation [7, 23]:

- cortex architectonics distortion (focal cortical dysplasia, foci of neuronal prolapse, and atrophy);
- reactive-destructive changes in cortical neurons (dystrophic changes of neurons, "shadow cells," satellitosis, and apoptosis);
- heterotopy of neurons into white matter;
- myelin damage and demyelination;

- rarefication of white matter and microcysts;
- sclerosis and dystonia of small vessels, angiomatosis;
- cellular astrocytic gliosis of white matter with oligodendroglia hyperplasia;
- hippocampal sclerosis with neuronal lesion and astrocytic gliosis.

3.2 Structural changes in the temporal lobe cortex

3.2.1 Focal cortical dysplasia (FCD)

Focal cortical dysplasia (FCD) is most often associated with structural DRE, including MR-negative or former cryptogenic. FCD is a type of cerebral cortex development disorder as a result of abnormal proliferation of neurons and glia, due to neuronal migration distortion and pathology of post-migration development [24–30]. They are characterized by a triad of histological signs [31]: disorders in the cerebral cortex layers formation (dyslamination) (type I), the presence of dysmorphic neurons and balloon cells (type II) (**Figure 4A, C,** and **D**). In addition, according to I. Blümcke et al., there are 2 more signs [32]: smoothness of the border between gray and white matter with the presence of a large number of heterotopic neurons in the white matter and myelination disorder in the adjacent white matter. Dyslamination to varying degrees always occurs with all variants of FCD but is especially pronounced with type I FCD. Dysmorphic neurons are characterized by

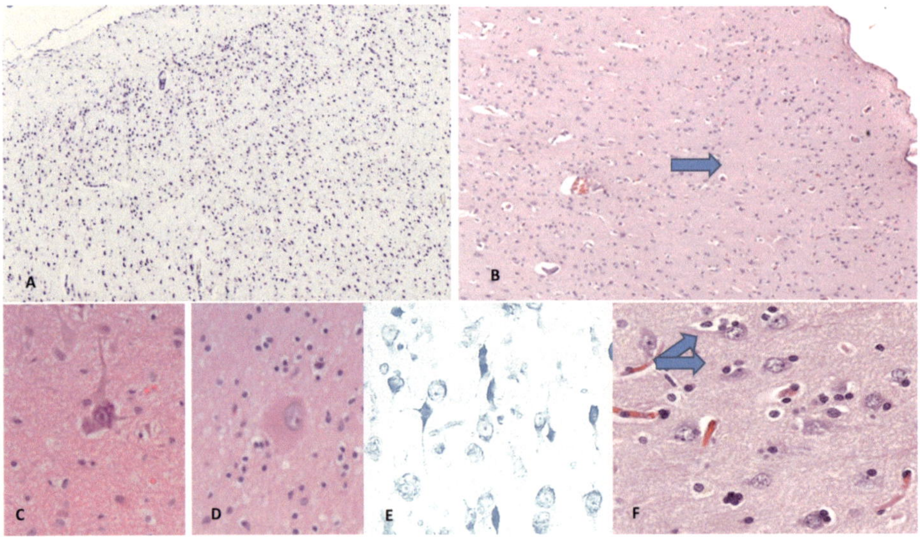

Figure 4.
Structural changes of the gray matter of the brain. A—Disorders of horizontal lamination and area of increased cellularity of the molecular layer. Nissl stain, x 100. B—Atrophic changes in the cortex: Disorders of architectonics with foci of neuronal prolapse (indicated by an arrow) and severe scalloped marginal layer of the cortex. H&E, x 100. C—Dysmorphic neuron (enlarged, with thickened processes, aggregation and displacement of the Nissl substance to the cell membrane. H&E, x 400. D—A large ballon cell with an opalescent "vitreous" cytoplasm with no Nissl substance. H&E, x 400. E—Most neurons are in a state of acute swelling with the phenomena of neuronophagy. Individual cells are in a state of wrinkling. Nissl stain, x 400. F—Ischemic changes in neurons, satellitosis, and neuronophagy (indicated by an arrow). H&E, x 400.

a significant increase in cell size, large cell nuclei; abnormal location of the Nissl substance (with a shift to the cell membrane); and accumulation of neurofilaments in the cytoplasm (type IIa) [32]. The presence of balloon cells is a distinctive feature of type IIb FCD. Balloon cells are found in all layers of the cortex (including layer I) and are represented by enlarged cells, often with the presence of several nuclei ("poly-nuclear" with "bridges" between them) and opalescent "vitreous" cytoplasm with the absence of Nissl substance [33].

Type III PCDs are a combination of cortical lamination disorders with other local pathological changes in the brain. The most common variant is a combination of cortical dysplasia with hippocampal sclerosis.

3.2.2 Reactive-destructive changes in cortical neurons

In the cortex, reactive-dystrophic and destructive changes of neurons are observed in nerve cells (**Figure 4E**). Neurons with hydropic dystrophy, chromatolysis, and vacuolization of the cytoplasm, alternate with hyperchromic shrunken cells. Among the altered neurons, "shadow cells" are identified that have retained the outlines of the cytoplasm with complete lysis of the nucleus. These changes are accompanied by moderately pronounced satellite disease and neuronophagy (**Figure 4F**). Reactive-destructive changes of neurons in the epileptic focus are accompanied by the ease of triggering membrane potentials, also contribute to the selective loss of GABA-ergic synaptic terminals, and are considered as morphological manifestations of partial neural deafferentation. In turn neural deafferentation causes hypersensitivity of cortical neurons to the perception of hypersynchronous discharges and determines increased spontaneous neural activity and sensitivity of synaptic receptors [34].

3.2.3 Foci of prolapse and atrophy of the cortex

In patients with DRE, all cases under study have demonstrated architectonic disturbances in the temporal lobe of the brain at the site of neuron death due to areas of complete loss of nerve cells and/or small-cell areas of small atrophied neurons and single gliocytes, as well as the phenomenon of cortical atrophy with a scalloped gyrus surface and a compacted neuropile of the I layer (**Figure 4B**).

3.3 Structural changes of white matter

3.3.1 Damage to the myelin sheath

In biopsies of patients with epilepsy with Spielmeyer staining for myelin, areas of weakly colored fibers, an indistinct border with the bark due to the depletion of fibers by myelin has been revealed (**Figure 5A–D**). During electron microscopic examination, significant damage to the myelin sheaths of axons is recorded, as manifested by myelin stratification, homogenization of its layers, and complete demyelination of axons. Most axons with damaged myelin sheaths retain their viability. This indicates that demyelination is not a secondary process and is not associated with the death of neurons and its processes. In addition, along with demyelination, depletion of the white matter by neurofilaments has been observed, that is, a decrease in the number of neuronal axons. Research data shows that the occurrence of epilepsy is associated with damage to the myelin sheath [23, 35–37]. Demyelination of fibers in the focus of epileptiform activity and adjacent pathways cause transverse neurotransmission and

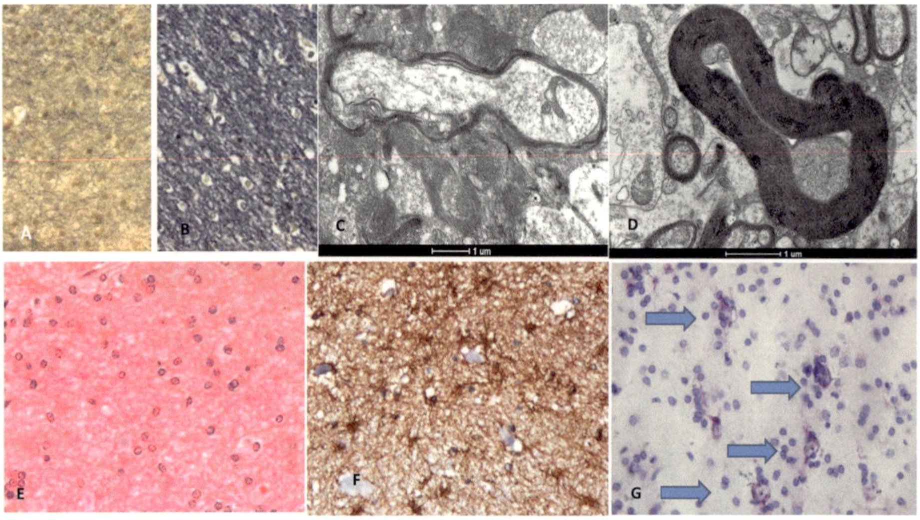

Figure 5.
Structural changes of white matter. A—White matter demyelination in a patient with DRE. Spielmeyer staining absent, × 200; B—Spielmeyer staining white matter rich in norm myelin. × 200; C—Longitudinal section of myelinated fiber with areas of granular myelin decay. Electronogram, × 16,500; D—Hypermyelination and destruction of the axial cylinder. Electronogram. × 20000; E—Increased cellularity of white matter due to glial elements (gliosis). H&E, x 400; F—Astrocytic gliosis. Immunohistochemistry with antibodies to GFAP, x 400; and G—Ectopic neurons (indicated by an arrow) among gliosis. Nissl stain, x 400.

generalization of nerve impulses with simultaneous involvement in epileptogenesis of various brain regions. Experimental studies have found that epilepsy reduces not only the amount of the main protein myelin but also the number of mature oligodendrocytes [35, 37].

3.3.2 Gliosis

Glial proliferation is considered to be a pathological substrate of epilepsy [38–40]. Gliosis is an integral part of the pathomorphological changes that are found in epileptic foci. Gliosis in the white matter is a uniform distribution of gliocytes with rounded stamped nuclei, and some cells have an optically empty cytoplasm, representing drainage forms of oligodendrogliocytes (**Figure 5E** and **F**). Immunohistochemical examination reveals clusters of intensely colored hypertrophied reactive astrocytes with pronounced processes.

Recent studies have revealed the involvement of electrical synapses (gap junction) in epileptogenesis, and it has been noted that the expression of the astrocytic protein connexin (connexin—C×43) is increased in patients with epilepsy associated with brain tumors and hippocampal sclerosis [41, 42].

The authors associated the increase in the amount of the C×43 protein with an increase in synaptic connections caused by intense electrochemical activity in "epileptic conditions." Thus, being not directly involved in the origin of paroxysmal discharges, the distribution patterns of C×43 protein can be involved in the development of (hyper) synchronization of neural discharges, providing a "short circuit" between electrically activated neurons, acting as "bridges" between different clusters of neural hyperexcitability, thus allowing the rapid spread of electrical activity [42, 43].

Clinical and morphological studies have recently proved that gliosis in DRE is not a pathological but an adaptive (protective) reaction: The more intense the proliferation of astrocytes, the milder the disease proceeds [44]. These data confirm the importance of glia in the pathogenesis of epilepsy. The research has shown that proliferation of oligodendroglial-like cells in epileptic foci can serve as a substrate for multifocal brain damage, which requires repeated resections. The specific neurophysiological mechanisms of excitability and epileptogenesis in oligodendroglial hyperplasia remain unclear since glial cells lack an action potential. Oligodendroglial hyperplasia may have direct or indirect effect on the population of subgranular cortical layer's neuronal cells with subsequent disruption of neural network activity and may represent an epiphenomenon due to repeated seizures from an unidentified focus [45].

3.3.3 Heterotopic neurons in the white matter

A typical morphological finding is heterotopic neurons in the subcortical zone. Random neurons of medium size, usually with the phenomena of hydropic dystrophy, are located in the deeper parts of the white matter (**Figure 5G**). A. Palmini et al. (2004) was introduced the term "mild developmental disorders of the cerebral cortex" due to the presence of a large number of clusters of heterotopic neurons located in the molecular layer of the cortex or in the subcortical white matter [29]. This persistent phenomenon is attributed to characteristic signs associated with FCD [32]. It is still unclear whether the density of heterotopic neurons in the white matter increases in patients with epilepsy and what the threshold for diagnostic confirmation of small cortical malformations should be [46], since the severity of these pathological signs correlates with preoperative MRI and is a clinically significant prognostic biomarker, in particular, for the result after surgery for epilepsy [47]. According to our data, in patients with epilepsy, the number of neurons in the white matter is significantly higher compared to other pathologies without epilepsy [7].

3.3.4 Microcystis

The white substance has a porous or microcystic structure (**Figure 6A–C**). There is a rarefication up to the microcystic transformation of white matter, the appearance of criblures with the expansion of spaces around the vessels. Thin collagen fibers are visible in the walls of some cysts. Electron microscopic examination revealed that the marginal zone of the cavities consists of three components. The distinctive feature of the internal component is its constant thickness (0.18–0.20 microns). It is represented by electron-dense material, in which fibrils are distinguishable. The main feature of the second (intermediate) component is a large number of collagen fibers. In some cases, they are visible even with light microscopy on preparations stained by the Van Gieson and Mallory methods. The outer component of the marginal zone is represented by edematous processes of astrocytes.

Damage to the vessels often causes the appearance of pseudocysts. However, they could develop in the outcome of inflammation and loss of myelin as well. In some cases, brain death can be assumed to occur due to ischemia and/or damage by blood plasma.

3.3.5 Angiopathy

Degenerative vascular changes are a typical phenomenon in the epileptic focus area. These are characterized by sclerosis or hyalinosis of the walls, formation of

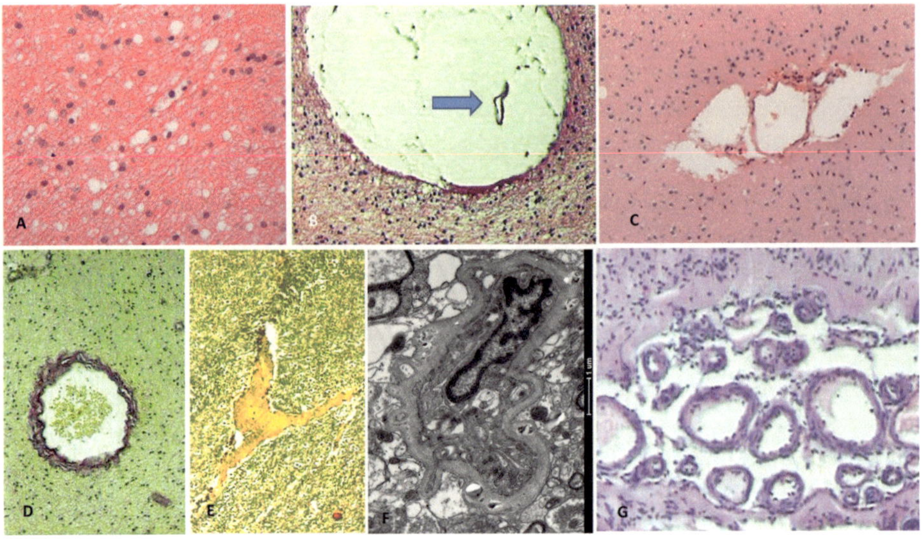

Figure 6.
Microcysts and angiopathy white matter. A—Microcystic transformation of white matter. H&E, x 400; B—Criblyura in white matter. A wide perivascular space forming a cavity. There is a small vessel in the lumen. H&E, x 200; C—Perivascular micro-cavity as a result of encephalolysis. H&E, x 200; D—A vessel with sclerosis thickened wall. Van Gieson stain, x 200; E—Dilated vein with uneven contours, with blood stasis. The sclerosed vein wall forms invaginates. Van Gieson stain, x 200; F—Unevenly thickened basement membrane of the spasmodic capillary. Electronogram. × 11500; and G—Foci of angiomatosis in the subarachnoid space. H&E, x 200.

convolutes and invaginates, and an increase in the diameter and wall stretching (**Figure 6D** and **E**).

Ultrastructural studies record damage to the capillary bed involving all elements of the blood-brain barrier (BBB) (**Figure 5F**). The nuclei of endotheliocytes are deformed and multilobed, and the cytoplasm is edematous. The basement membrane loses the clarity of contours, becomes loose, and uneven in thickness, marked by delamination and vacuolization foci. The perivascular coupling is represented by edematous processes of astrocytes, and many fragments of capillaries are completely devoid of it. In these zones, myelinated axons with significantly damaged myelin are closely attached to the vessels.

There were signs of restructuring the vascular bed with the formation of foci of angiomatosis. The changes detected are attributed to the consequences of chronic hemodynamic disorders, aggravating hypoxia in the tissues, which in turn contributes to the development of convulsive states.

3.4 Hippocampal sclerosis

Hippocampal sclerosis is a common morphological substrate in temporal lobe epilepsy and is characterized by hippocampus cellular structure disorders, that is, neuronal death and gliosis [32, 33, 48]. Although the generally accepted meaning of "sclerosis" (from the Greek word *scleros*—seal) is the sealing of an organ with the replacement of parenchymal cells by connective tissue, in the pathology of the nervous system, it also implies gliosis [49]. This phenomenon is also called mesial temporal sclerosis, incisural sclerosis, or "Ammon's horn sclerosis" [50]. Along with the death of neurons and proliferation of glia in hippocampal sclerosis, dispersion of granular cells of the dentate gyrus is detected [51]. It is characterized by the expansion of the granular layer, the separation of cells from each other with a violation of the compact dense structure, and their spread into the molecular layer (**Figure 7**). The presence of hippocampal sclerosis and extra-hippocampal pathology is called "dual pathology," which occurs in 5–34% of cases of temporal lobe epilepsy [50, 52].

However, in addition to structural changes in the hippocampal formation, functional ones are also distinguished, which include loss of GABAergic neurons, lack of reelin, axonal springing of mossy fibers, and neurogenesis. Loss of hippocampal neurons can also be observed in other pathological conditions, including neurodegeneration, aging, and ischemia, but the nature of neuronal loss varies significantly [53] and usually affects the subiculum [54, 55].

While the pathogenesis of hippocampal sclerosis is still a controversial and unclear issue, the role of the hippocampus in the development of medial temporal epilepsy is obvious. The normal cytoarchitectonics of the hippocampus, the density of neurons in it, and their unidirectional spatial orientation create conditions for hyperexcitability along synaptic and extra-synaptic ephaptic pathways [5]. According to experimental data, the hippocampal formation has the lowest threshold of convulsive readiness, 10 times lower than that of the sensorimotor cortex [56]. It was previously assumed that the death of neurons, cellular reorganization, and glial proliferation in the hippocampus during its sclerosis lead to increased excitability of granular cells of the dentate gyrus, which spreads from the hippocampus and generates an epileptic seizure [57]. The death of inhibitory interneurons, the formation of synapses, and the proliferation (springing) of mossy fibers of excitatory neurons can also lead to the formation of a focus of hyperactivity. Some authors believe that the growth (springing) of mossy fibers is a compensatory-restorative process [58].

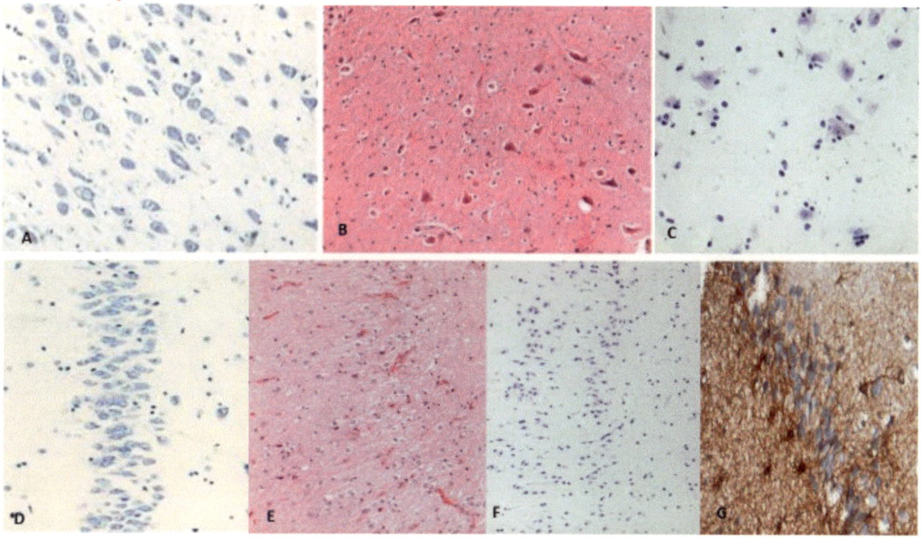

Figure 7.
Hippocampal sclerosis. A—The nucleus of the hippocampus, without significant changes. Nissl stain, x 200; B—Severe disorders of cytoarchitectonics, atrophic changes in the form of foci of prolapse of neurons in the nuclei of the hippocampus, up to the emptying of structures. H&E x 200; C—Preserved neurons with the phenomena of satellite disease. Nissl stain, x 400; D—Dentate gyrus without significant changes. Nissl stain, x 200; E—Dispersion of the granular layer of the dentate gyrus. H&E, x 200; F—Bifurcation of the granular layer of the dentate gyrus. Nissl stain, x 200; and G—Astrocytic glial proliferation in the dentate gyrus. Immunohistochemistry with antibodies to GFAP, x 400.

Comparison of the two groups (with and without epilepsy) against the totality of the neuron density values and glia cellularity allows us to state that the hippocampus in patients with DRE is a homogeneous cluster, regardless of the degree of morphological changes, which indicates the formation of a specific "epileptic" hippocampus in this category of patients [59].

While the epileptic system is being formed, the hippocampus can act as a "generator" of increased arousal, the primary focus of epilepticism, and can also be involved in the process of epilepticism of the brain as a result of triggering extra-hippocampal forms of the disease.

4. Glioneuronal apoptosis

Astrocytes are known to play an important role in epileptogenesis [60–62]. Astrocyte apoptosis is assumed to activate during and after a convulsive attack and may contribute to neuronal death and epileptogenesis [63]. Our studies have demonstrated that apoptosis can be observed mainly in oligodendrocytes, single astrocytes, and a small part of neurons only (**Figure 8**) [40, 64, 65].

A study on rat oligodendrocyte culture showed that oligodendrocyte apoptosis in the epilepsy model was higher than in the control one [66]. There is evidence that NK cells can induce apoptosis in both neurons and mature oligodendrocytes via the FAS-FAS-L pathway [67]. The main function of oligodendrocytes is the formation of axon myelin sheaths. In epilepsy, the number of mature oligodendrocytes and the

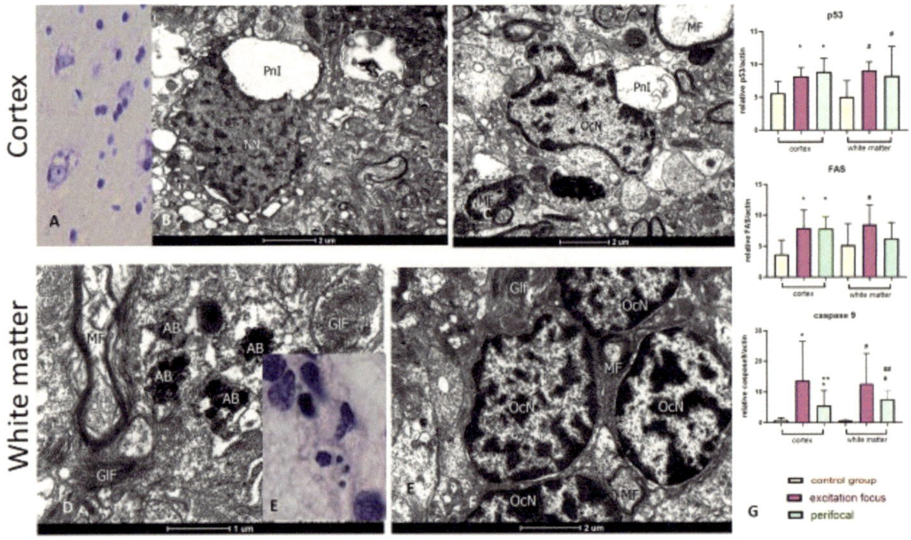

Figure 8.
*Glioneuronal apoptosis in the epileptic focus of the temporal lobe. A—Destructive changes in neurons (deformation of the nuclei, pronounced vacuolization, and local cytoplasmic tigroid). Increase in the number of glial cells. Nissl staining, ×400; B—Vacuoles and perinuclear inflation in an apoptotic neuron (N); ×8200; C—Perinuclear inflation in the oligodendrocyte; ×8200; D—Apoptotic bodies in the intercellular space;×16,500; E—Apoptotic bodies in the white matter of the brain. Nissl staining, ×1000. Immersion; F—The initial stage of apoptosis. An accumulation of oligodendrocytes in the white matter of the brain, the heterochromatin of which is distributed throughout the nucleus in large conglomerates. OcN: Oligodendrocyte nucleus, GlF: Gliofibrils, MF: Myelin fibers; ×8200; and G—Histogram of the content of proapoptotic proteins in cortical and white matter biopsies of patients with DRE compared to control group patients. *Cortex, p<0.05; #white matter, p<0.05. Electronogram—B, C, D, and F.*

amount of myelin decreases [35]. In the hippocampus of rats, the loss of myelin and oligodendrocytes begins in the acute phase and progresses in the latent and chronic phases of epileptogenesis [68].

The survival of oligodendrocytes depends on many factors, including the condition of astrocytes, which secrete growth factors important for the survival of neurons, glia, and glial proliferation [7]. The loss of oligodendrocytes leads to an imbalance of excitation and inhibition in the brain and provokes the formation of an epileptic focus or exacerbates the severity of epilepsy [35].

5. Neuroinflammation

5.1 The cytokine levels in blood plasma in drug-resistant epilepsy

According to experimental and clinical data, DRE is characterized by the presence of neuroinflammation in an epileptogenic focus [69]. Glial cells, such as astrocytes and microglia, produce and release cytokines and chemokines, which play an important role in the development of chronic neuroinflammation in epilepsy [70]. Cytokines can have both pro- and anticonvulsant activity, acting on AMPA and NMDA receptors and having a neurotoxic effect. Detecting cytokines such as TNF-α, IL-1, and IL-8 in the blood typically indicates acute inflammation. Their effects are regulated by the pro-inflammatory IFN-γ, IL-12, and inflammatory inhibitors, such as IL-10, expressed in response. We studied the cytokine levels in blood plasma samples of DRE patients (multiplex analysis). However, our results demonstrate a normal level of the studied cytokines, except for an increased level of TNF-α and insufficient IL-2. IL-2 is known to promote the regeneration of neurons after their damage, and also stimulates the proliferation and differentiation of oligodendrogliocytes. The revealed insufficient level of IL-2 may be one of the reasons for the decrease in the bioavailability of therapeutic drugs, depending on the function of the blood-brain barrier (BBB). BBB changes in many pathologies of the central nervous system, including activation of adhesion molecules in the vascular lumen, increased adhesion and transmigration of leukocytes, increased permeability of tight contacts, and extravasation of plasma proteins [71]. Earlier experimental and clinical studies have found that BBB permeability increases in foci of long-term epilepsy, and artificially induced BBB dysfunction leads to the appearance of epileptic foci in previously healthy brains [72, 73].

IL-4 is involved in balancing neuroinflammation. Our data showed an increase in IL-4 levels, which may indicate its response to the appearance of TNF-α in the blood. An increase in IL-4 levels may be compensatory for slowing down the synthesis of cytokines of the primary response [74]. The reduced level of IL-8 detected by us may contribute to increased adhesion of neutrophils activated by pro-inflammatory cytokines to endothelial cells. This is how endothelial damage and increased BBB permeability occur [74]. Astrocytes secrete chemokines (EGF, TGF-β, and VEGF), which directly affect endothelial cells. The high content of chemokines in the blood of DRE patients indicates the activation of astrocytes and the negative effect of neuroinflammation on the BBB [75].

5.2 The expression of cytokines in neural tissue in DRE

The study of the content of pro-inflammatory cytokines in the epileptogenic focus itself and its perifocal zone allowed us to assess the course and degree of neuroinflammation depending on their epileptogenic activity. Our study showed the presence of neuroinflammation and apoptosis in brain tissues. The content of pro and antiapoptotic proteins and pro-inflammatory cytokines (p-NF-kB, TNF-α, p53, FAS, caspase-3, caspase-9, etc.) was analyzed in biopsies of gray and white matter of the temporal lobe of the brain of DRE patients obtained intraoperatively (Western blotting). In the cortex and white matter of the perifocal zone, an increased content of proapoptotic proteins (TNF-α, p53, FAS, caspase-3, caspase-9) has been found against an imbalance of protective pathway proteins (p-NF-kB—p. 65 and p. 105). In the epileptic focus, the process of neuroinflammation prevails over the process of apoptosis. In the samples we took, an increased content of TNF-α cytokine was detected both in the epileptic focus and in the perifocal zone of the focus in the cortex and white matter of the temporal lobe of the brain. Similarly, increased expression of the FAS receptor was observed in the epileptic focus of gray and white matter of the temporal lobe as compared with the values of the control group. In the perifocal zone of the epileptic focus, the expression of FAS was increased only in the cortex, while an upward trend was observed in the white matter. The high content of TNF-α has been found in biopsies of the cortex and white matter of the temporal lobe against the increased expression of the FAS-L receptor, which may indicate activation of immune cells in the brain of DRE patients and neuroinflammatory processes in these areas. In the perifocal zone, these processes may occur as well, however, less intensively [76].

Pro-inflammatory cytokines are known to grow in number during seizures, which increases the excitability of neurons and results in recurrent seizures, cell death, and inflammation development [77].

Thus, epileptic seizures, accompanied by neuroinflammation and apoptosis with blood-brain barrier distortion in the background, have a mutually provoking effect and contribute to pathological process to be sustained (**Figure 9**).

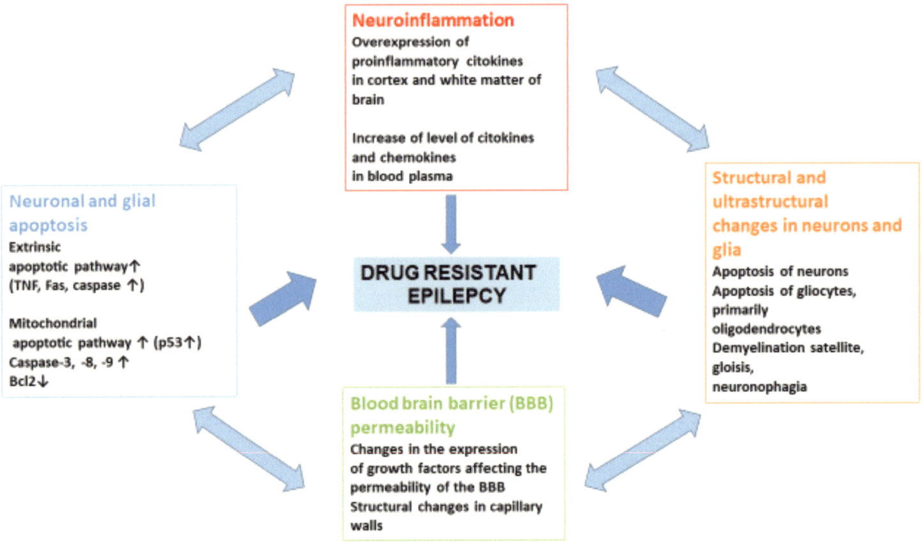

Figure 9.
Pathogenesis of drug-resistant epilepsy (scheme).

6. Epileptic leukoencephalopathy

Changes in brain tissue and its membranes are nonspecific, but the complexity of these nonspecific processes creates a morphological picture of damage and compensatory adaptive processes characteristic of epilepsy. Significant changes are observed in the white matter. Demyelination, angiopathy, and microcysts of white matter, as well as cellular gliosis, which are usually described in epileptic foci, were qualified by O.N. Gaykova (2001) as the syndrome of "epileptic leukoencephalopathy" [23]. This was the first step toward a syndrome approach in the clinical and pathomorphological characterization of epilepsy. Radical structural changes in the white matter in DRE are a zone characterized by discharge and microcystic transformation as a result of cell death, demyelination as a result of repeated seizures, increasing hypoxia with the angiopathy in background, and the blood-brain barrier distortion. The loss of substance in an epileptic focus with reactive astrocyte proliferation is qualified as a parenchymal atrophy of the brain and may already serve as an epileptogenic focus (**Figure 10**).

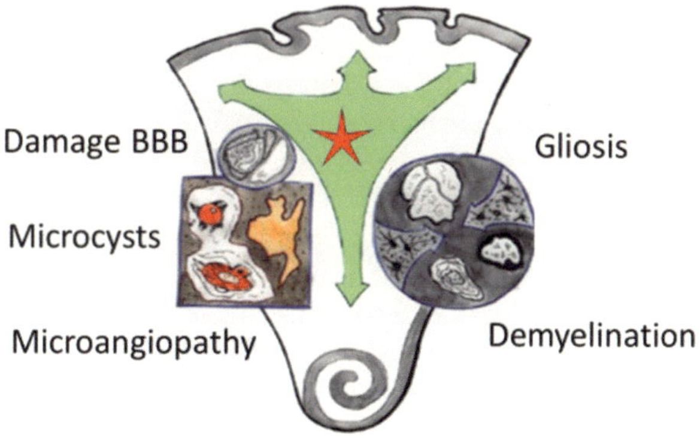

Figure 10.
The epileptogenic role of the structural lesion of white matter (leukoencephalopathy) in the epileptic focus (scheme) (author's drawing by professor O.N Gaikova [78]).

7. Conclusions

The research data demonstrate the heterogeneity and complexity of etiopathogenetic interactions representing the morphogenesis of structural changes detected in the epileptic activity zone (epileptic focus), as a stable epileptic system is forming. The area of epileptic foci in DRE is characterized by the depletion of white matter with myelin and neuronal processes, replaced by astrocytic gliosis and manifested in rarefaction of the neuropile with parenchymal or/and perivascular cystic transformation of brain tissue leading to the formation of epileptic leukoencephalopathy, which in itself can be qualified as epileptogenic focus. Neuronal and oligodendroglial apoptosis in combination with neuroinflammation form a self-sustaining pathological focus, which leads to the progression of the disease and the occurrence of relapses. Reactive-destructive processes in the hippocampus with an outcome in atrophy and the hippocampus sclerosis reveal specific features and can also be qualified as the structural basis of the drug-resistant epileptic system and can become a factor of epilepticism. In addition, the revealed insufficiency of compensatory and adaptive mechanisms, including glio- and neurogenesis, can ensure the progression of the process and be accompanied by a decrease in sensitivity to drug therapy.

The authors propose the conception of the epileptic focus on heterogeneous structural organization in DRE, which allows qualifying the epileptic focus as a complex structural and functional system with elements of biochemical and mediator processes being distorted, featuring numerous mutually potentiating epileptogenic and supporting epileptic system interactions, and characterized by insufficient compensatory and adaptive mechanisms that ensure the progression of the process, accompanied by a decrease in sensitivity to drug therapy [7].

The conceptual approach to heterogeneous structural organization of epileptic foci in DRE opens up prospects for developing a treatment strategy aiming to break the pathological circle by identifying the targets for therapeutic effects, including possible local lifetime mutations and gene expression.

Acknowledgements

We express our deep gratitude to the teachers—professors of the Polenov Russian Scientific Research Institute of Neurosurgery—Yuri V. Zotov, Yuri A. Medvedev, Sergey L Yatsuk, Tamara S. Stepanova, who influenced our scientific views and clinical experience.

We thank the neurosurgeons and neurologists of the Polenov Institute involved in the treatment of epilepsy patients who helped in the creation of this chapter.

The work was supported by the Russian Foundation for Basic Research (project No. 20-015-00127) and the state task of the National Almazov Medical Research Center No. 056-00109-21-01(19). TEM (FEITecnai G2Spirit BioTWIN, Netherlands), provided by Collective Equipment Center of Sechenov Institute of Evolutionary Physiology and Biochemistry, Russian Academy of Sciences.

Conflict of interest

The authors declare no conflict of interest.

Abbreviations

DRE	drug-resistant epilepsy
EEG	electroencephalography
ECoG	electrocorticography
EsubCoG	electrosubcorticography
FCD	focal cortical dysplasia
BBB	blood-brain barrier

Author details

Yulia M. Zabrodskaya[1], Olga N. Gaykova[2], Mikhail V. Alexandrov[1], Natalia M. Paramonova[3,4], Darya A. Sitovskaya[1,5]*, Anastasya V. Litovchenko[3], Tatiana V. Sokolova[1], Sofiia E. Cherenkova[1] and Elena D. Bazhanova[2,3,6]

1 Polenov Neurosurgical Institute—Branch of the Almazov National Medical Research Centre, St. Petersburg, Russia

2 Golikov Research Center of Toxicology, St. Petersburg, Russia

3 Sechenov Institute of Evolutionary Physiology and Biochemistry, Russian Academy of Sciences, St. Petersburg, Russia

4 State Research Testing Institute of Military Medicine of the Ministry of Defense of the Russian Federation, St. Petersburg, Russia

5 St. Petersburg State Pediatric Medical University, St. Petersburg, Russia

6 Astrakhan State University, Astrakhan, Russia

*Address all correspondence to: daliya_16@mail.ru

References

[1] Ravizza T, Terrone G, Salamone A, Frigerio F, Balosso S, Antoine DJ, et al. High mobility group box 1 is a novel pathogenic factor and a mechanistic biomarker for epilepsy. Brain, Behavior, and Immunity. 2018;**72**:14-21. DOI: 10.1016/j.bbi.2017.10.008. Epub 2017 Oct 13

[2] Bernhardt BC, Hong SJ, Bernasconi A, Bernasconi N. Magnetic resonance imaging pattern learning in temporal lobe epilepsy: Classification and prognostics. Annals of Neurology. 2015;**77**(3):436-446. DOI: 10.1002/ana.24341. Epub 2015 Jan 13

[3] Neligan A, Hauser WA, Sander JW. The epidemiology of the epilepsies. Handbook of Clinical Neurology. 2012;**107**:113-133. DOI: 10.1016/B978-0-444-52898-8.00006-9

[4] Aivazyan SO, Lukyanova EG, Shiryaev YS. Modern treatment options for drug-resistant epilepsy in children. Epilepsy and Paroxysmal Conditions. 2014;**6**(1):34-43. (In Russ.)

[5] Karlov VA. Epilepsy in Children and Adult Men and Women. Moscow: Meditsina; 2010. p. 717. (In Russ.)

[6] Sommer W. Die Erkrankung des Ammons horn salsa etiologisches Moment der Epilepsie. Arch. Psychiat. Nervenkr. 1880;**308**:631-675

[7] Sitovskaya DA, Zabrodskaya YM, SokolovaTV,KuralbaevAK,NezdorovinaVG, Dobrogorskaya LN. Strukturnaya geterogennost' epilepticheskikh ochagov pri lokal'noi farmakorezistentnoi epilepsii [Structural heterogeneity of epileptic foci in local drug-resistant epilepsy]. Arkh Patol. 2020;**82**(6):5-15. DOI: 10.17116/patol2020820615. (Russian)

[8] Aleksandrov MV, Ivanov LB, Lytaev SA, et al. Electroencephalography. Guidelines. 2019. p. 224. (In Russ.)

[9] Luders HO, editor. Textbook of Epilepsy Surgery. London: CRC Press; 2008. p. 1648

[10] Aleksandrov MV, Chikurov AA, Toporkova OA, et al. In: Alexandrov MV, editor. Neurophysiological Intraoperative Monitoring in Neurosurgery: A Guide. 2nd ed., revised and expanded. Saint Petersburg: SpetsLit; 2020. p. 159. (In Russ.)

[11] Krylov VV. In: Krylov VV, editor. Epilepsy Surgery / [Collection]. Moscow: ABV-press; 2019. p. 400. (In Russ.)

[12] Astakhova EA, Cherenkova SE, Marchenko EV, Sebelev KI, Aleksandrov MV. The relationship of bioelectric activity and structural changes in the hippocampus at pharmacoresistant temporal lobe epilepsy. Translational Medicine. 2021;**8**(2):5-13. (In Russ.). DOI: 10.18705/2311-4495-2021-8-2-5-13

[13] Wang Z, Larivière S, Xu Q, Vos de Wael R, Hong SJ, Wang Z, et al. Community-informed connectomics of the thalamocortical system in generalized epilepsy. Neurology. 2019;**93**(11):e1112-e1122. DOI: 10.1212/WNL.0000000000008096. Epub 2019 Aug 12

[14] Curia G, Lucchi C, Vinet J, Gualtieri F, Marinelli C, Torsello A, et al. Pathophysiogenesis of mesial temporal lobe epilepsy: Is prevention of damage antiepileptogenic? Current Medicinal Chemistry. 2014;**21**(6):663-688. DOI: 10.2174/0929867320666131119152201

[15] Labate A, Aguglia U, Tripepi G, Mumoli L, Ferlazzo E, Baggetta R, et al. Long-term outcome of mild mesial temporal lobe epilepsy: A prospective longitudinal cohort study. Neurology. 2016;**86**(20):1904-1910. DOI: 10.1212/WNL.0000000000002674. Epub 2016 Apr 20

[16] Barbaro NM, Quigg M, Ward MM, Chang EF, Broshek DK, Langfitt JT, et al. Radiosurgery versus open surgery for mesial temporal lobe epilepsy: The randomized, controlled ROSE trial. Epilepsia. 2018;**59**(6):1198-1207. DOI: 10.1111/epi.14045. Epub 2018 Mar 30

[17] Aleksandrov MV, Kostenko IA, Arkhipova NB, Basharin VA, Tolkach PG, Chernyi VS, et al. Suppression of brain electrical activity in general anesthesia: The dose-effect relationship. Bulletin of the Russian Military Medical Academy. 2018;**20**(4):79-85. DOI: 10.17816/brmma12279

[18] Miller RD. In: Miller RD, editor. Miller's Anesthesia. Churchill, Livingstone: Elsevier; 2005. p. 3576

[19] Thijs RD, Surges R, O'Brien TJ, Sander JW. Epilepsy in adults. Lancet. 2019;**393**(10172):689-701. DOI: 10.1016/S0140-6736(18)32596-0. Epub 2019 Jan 24

[20] Cherenkova SE, Tastanbekov MM, Nazarov RV, Aleksandrov MV. Monitoring of the bioelectrical activity of the hippocampal complex: the effect of inhalation anesthetics as a functional test. Medical Alphabet. 2021;**28**:16-22. DOI: 10.33667/2078-5631-2021-28-16-22. (In Russ.)

[21] Lahl R, Villagran R, Teixeira W. Neuropathology of Focal Epilepsies: An Atlas. Bielefeld: John Libbey and Co. Ltd; 2003. p. 320. DOI: 10.1111/j.0013-9580.2004.20404.x

[22] Meencke HJ, Janz D. Neuropathological findings in primary generalized epilepsy: A study of eight cases. Epilepsia. 1984;**25**(1):8-21. DOI: 10.1111/j.1528-1157.1984.tb04149.x

[23] Gaikova ON, Suvorov AV, Paramonova NM. Significance of cerebral white matter damage in pathogenesis of localization related epilepsy. Rossiiskii neirokhirurgicheskii zhurnal imeni professora a.L. Polenova/Russian Neurosurgical Journal named after professor A.L. Polenov. 2011;**3**(1):19-24. (In Russ.)

[24] Alikhanov AA, Nikanorov AY, Mukhin KY, Ayvazyan SO. Focal cortical dysplasia in patient with epileptic seizures. Zhurnal nevrologii i psikhiatrii im. S.S. Korsakova (S.S. Korsakov Journal of Neurology and Psychiatry). 1998;**7**: 45-47. (In Russ.)

[25] Alikhanov AA, Petrukhin AS, Kyu M, et al. Magnetic resonance imaging with high resolution in the evaluation of epileptogenic brain lesions. Russkiy zhurnal detskoy nevrologii (Russian Journal of Child Neurology). 2006;**1**(1): 18-24. (In Russ.)

[26] Blümcke I. In: Shorvon S, Guerrini R, Cook M, Lhatoo S, editors. Developmental Neurobiology, Neuroanatomy and Neuropathology of Epilepsy. In: Oxford Textbook of Epilepsy and Epileptic Seizures. USA: Oxford University Press; 2013. pp. 39-50. DOI: 10.1093/med/9780199659043.003.0004

[27] Holthausen H, Piper T, Winkler P, et al. Electro-clinical-pathological correlations in focal cortical dysplasia (FCD) at young ages. Child's Nervous System. 2014;**30**(12):2015-2026. DOI: 10.1007/s00381-014-2549-6

[28] Sarnat HB, Blümcke I. In: Blümcke I, Sarnat HB, Coras R, editors. Malformations of Cortical Development. In: Surgical Neuropathology of Focal Epilepsies: Textbook and Atlas. Paris: John LibbeyEurotext; 2015. p. 160. DOI: 10.1093/jnen/nlw006

[29] Palmini A, Najm I, Avanzini G, Babb T, Guerrini R, Foldvary-Schaefer N, et al. Terminology and classification of the cortical dysplasias. Neurology. 2004;**62**(6 Suppl 3):S2-S8. DOI: 10.1212/01.wnl.0000114507.30388.7e

[30] Barkovich AJ, Guerrini R, Kuzniecky RI, Jackson GD, Dobyns WB. A developmental and genetic classification for malformations of cortical development: Update 2012. Brain. 2012;**135**(Pt 5):1348-1369. DOI: 10.1093/brain/aws019. Epub 2012 Mar 16

[31] Kuzniecky R. Focal cortical dysplasia and related variants. In: Shorvon S, Andermann F, Guerrini R, editors. The Causes of Epilepsy: Common and Uncommon Causes in Adults and Children. Cambridge: Cambridge University Press. pp. 293-297. DOI: 10.1017/CBO9780511921001.047

[32] Blümcke I, Thom M, Aronica E, et al. The clinic-pathologic spectrum of focal cortical dysplasias: A consensus classification proposed by an ad hoc task force of the ILAE diagnostic methods commission. Epilepsia. 2011;**52**(1):158-174. DOI: 10.1111/j.1528-1167.2010.02777.x

[33] Wieser H-G, editor. ILAE Commission Report. Mesial temporal lobe epilepsy with hippocampal sclerosis. ILAE Commission on Neurosurgery of Epilepsy // Epilepsia. 2004;**45**(6):695-714. DOI: 10.1007/springerreference_188282

[34] Karlov VA. Sudorozhnyi Epilepticheskii Status. M: MED press in form; 2003. p. 168. (InRuss.)

[35] Hu X, Wang JY, Gu R, Qu H, Li M, Chen L, et al. The relationship between the occurrence of intractable epilepsy with glial cells and myelin sheath—An experimental study. European Review for Medical and Pharmacological Sciences. 2016;**20**(21):4516-4524

[36] Lapato AS, Szu JI, Hasselmann JPC, et al. Chronic demyelination-induced seizures. Neuroscience. 2017;**27**(346):409-422. DOI: 10.1016/j.neuroscience.2017.01.035

[37] Kim SH, Choi J. Pathological classification of focal cortical dysplasia (FCD): Personal comments for well understanding FCD classification. Journal of Korean Neurosurgical Association. 2019;**62**(3):288-295. DOI: 10.3340/jkns.2019.0025. Epub 2019 May 1

[38] Devinsky O, Vezzani A, Najjar S, De Lanerolle NC, Rogawski MA. Glia and epilepsy: Excitability and inflammation. Trends in Neurosciences. 2013;**36**(3):174-184. DOI: 10.1016/j.tins.2012.11.008. Epub 2013 Jan 5

[39] Novozhilova AP, Gaikova ON. Cell gliosis of a white substance of the human brain and its significance in the pathogenesis of focal epilepsy. Morphology. 2001;**2**:20-24. (In Russ.)

[40] Sokolova TV, Zabrodskaya YM, Paramonova NM, Dobrogorskaya LN, Kuralbaev AK, Kasumov VR, et al. Apoptosis of brain cells in epileptic focus at phapmacresistant temporal lobe epilepsy. Translyatsionnaya Meditsina (Translational Medicine). 2017;**4**(6):22-33. (In Russ.)

[41] Aronica E, Gorter JA, Jansen GH, Leenstra S, Yankaya B, Troost D. Expression of connexin 43 and connexin 32 gap-junction proteins in epilepsy-associated brain tumors and in the

perilesional epileptic cortex. Acta Neuropathologica. 2001;**101**(5):449-459. DOI: 10.1007/s004010000305

[42] Fonseca CG, Green CR, Nicholson LF. Upregulation in astrocytic connexin 43 gap junction levels may exacerbate generalized seizures in mesial temporal lobe epilepsy. Brain Research. 2002;**929**(1):105-116. DOI: 10.1016/s0006-8993(01)03289-9

[43] Tassi L, Garbelli R, Colombo N, Bramerio M, Russo GL, Mai R, et al. Electroclinical, MRI and surgical outcomes in 100 epileptic patients with type II FCD. Epileptic Disorders. 2012;**14**(3):257-266. DOI: 10.1684/epd.2012.0525

[44] Medvedev YV, Bersnev VP, Kasumov VR, et al. Effect of the degree of severity of brain gliosis on the severity of the course of the disease in patients with medically resistant forms of locally caused epilepsy. Neurosurgery. 2010;**4**:65-90 (In Russ.)

[45] Henshall DC, Engel T. Contribution of apoptosis-associated signaling pathways to epileptogenesis: Lessons from Bcl-2 family knockouts. Frontiers in Cellular Neuroscience. 2013;**7**:110. DOI: 10.3389/fncel.2013.00110

[46] Schurr J, Coras R, Rössler K, Pieper T, Kudernatsch M, Holthausen H, et al. Mild malformation of cortical development with Oligodendroglial hyperplasia in frontal lobe epilepsy: A new Clinico-pathological entity. Brain Pathology. 2017;**27**(1):26-35. DOI: 10.1111/bpa.12347. Epub 2016 Feb 22

[47] Blümcke I, Aronica E, Miyata H, Sarnat HB, Thom M, Roessler K, et al. International recommendation for a comprehensive neuropathologic workup of epilepsy surgery brain tissue: A consensus task force report from the ILAE commission on diagnostic methods. Epilepsia. 2016;**57**(3):348-358. DOI: 10.1111/epi.13319. Epub 2016 Feb 3

[48] Blümcke I, Thom M, Wiestler OD. Ammon's horn sclerosis: A maldevelopmental disorder associated with temporal lobe epilepsy. Brain Pathology. 2002;**12**(2):199-211. DOI: 10.1111/j.1750-3639.2002.tb00436.x

[49] Sarkisov DS. Regeneration and its Clinical Significance. Hindawi: Medicina; 1970. p. 284. (In Russ.)

[50] Al Sufiani F, Ang LC. Neuropathology of temporal lobe epilepsy. Epilepsy Research and Treatment. 2012;**2012**:624519. DOI: 10.1155/2012/624519. Epub 2012 Apr 12

[51] Houser CR. Granule cell dispersion in the dentate gyrus of humans with temporal lobe epilepsy. Brain Research. 1990;**535**(2):195-204. DOI: 10.1016/0006-8993(90)91601-c

[52] Tassi L, Meroni A, Deleo F, Villani F, Mai R, Russo GL, et al. Temporal lobe epilepsy: Neuropathological and clinical correlations in 243 surgically treated patients. Epileptic Disorders. 2009;**11**(4):281-292. DOI: 10.1684/epd.2009.0279. Epub 2009 Nov 30

[53] Miyata H, Hori T, Vinters HV. Surgical pathology of epilepsy-associated non-neoplastic cerebral lesions: A brief introduction with special reference to hippocampal sclerosis and focal cortical dysplasia. Neuropathology. 2013;**33**(4):442-458. DOI: 10.1111/neup.12028. Epub 2013 Mar 27

[54] Nelson PT, Head E, Schmitt FA, Davis PR, Neltner JH, Jicha GA, et al. Alzheimer's disease is not "brain aging": Neuropathological, genetic, and epidemiological human studies.

Acta Neuropathologica. 2011;**121**(5): 571-587. DOI: 10.1007/s00401-011-0826-y. Epub 2011 Apr 24

[55] Montine TJ, Phelps CH, Beach TG, Bigio EH, Cairns NJ, Dickson DW, et al. Hyman BT; National Institute on Aging; Alzheimer's association. National Institute on Aging-Alzheimer's Association guidelines for the neuropathologic assessment of Alzheimer's disease: A practical approach. Acta Neuropathologica. 2012;**123**(1):1-11. DOI: 10.1007/s00401-011-0910-3. Epub 2011 Nov 20

[56] Zenkov LR. Klinicheskaya epileptologiya. Moskva: Med in form Agenstvo; 2010. p. 408. (In Russ.)

[57] von Campe G, Spencer DD, de Lanerolle NC. Morphology of dentate granule cells in the human epileptogenic hippocampus. Hippocampus. 1997;**7**(5):472-488. DOI: 10.1002/(SICI)1098-1063(1997)7:5<472::AID-HIPO4>3.0.CO;2-J

[58] Sutula TP, Dudek FE. Unmasking recurrent excitation generated by mossy fiber sprouting in the epileptic dentate gyrus: An emergent property of a complex system. Progress in Brain Research. 2007;**163**:541-563. DOI: 10.1016/S0079-6123(07)63029-5

[59] Sitovskaya DA, Semenov KK, Moshchenko SS, Sokolova TV, Zabrodskaya YM. Cellular imbalance of the hippocampus in drug-resistant epilepsy (on the role of the hippocampus in epileptogenesis). Rossiiskii neirokhirurgicheskii zhurnal imeni professora A.L. Polenova/Russian Neurosurgical Journal named after professor A.L. Polenov. 2022;**14**(3):80-88. DOI: 10.56618/20712693_2022_14_3_80 (In Russ.)

[60] Bedner P, Dupper A, Hüttmann K, Müller J, Herde MK, Dublin P, et al. Astrocyte uncoupling as a cause of human temporal lobe epilepsy. Brain. 2015;**138**(Pt 5):1208-1222. DOI: 10.1093/brain/awv067. Epub 2015 Mar 12

[61] Narkilahti S, Pirttilä TJ, Lukasiuk K, Tuunanen J, Pitkänen A. Expression and activation of caspase 3 following status epilepticus in the rat. The European Journal of Neuroscience. 2003;**18**(6):1486-1496. DOI: 10.1046/j.1460-9568.2003.02874.x

[62] Henshall DC, Simon RP. Epilepsy and apoptosis pathways. Journal of Cerebral Blood Flow and Metabolism. 2005;**25**(12):1557-1572. DOI: 10.1038/sj.jcbfm.9600149

[63] Engel T, Henshall DC. Apoptosis, Bcl-2 family proteins and caspases: The ABCs of seizure-damage and epileptogenesis? International Journal of Physiology, Pathophysiology and Pharmacology. 2009;**1**(2):97-115

[64] Sazhina TA, Sitovskaya DA, Zabrodskaya YM, et al. Functional imbalance of glutamate- and GABAergic neuronal Systems in the Pathogenesis of focal drug-resistant epilepsy in humans. Bulletin of Experimental Biology and Medicine. 2020;**168**(4):529-532. DOI: 10.1007/s10517-020-04747-3

[65] Litovchenko AV, Zabrodskaya YM, Sitovskaya DA, et al. Markers of neuroinflammation and apoptosis in the temporal lobe of patients with drug-resistent epilepsy. Journal of Evolutionary Biochemistry and Physiology. 2021;**57**(5):1040-1049. DOI: 10.1134/S0022093021050069

[66] Luo X, Li Z, Zhao J, Deng Y, Zhong Y, Zhang M. Fyn gene silencing reduces oligodendrocytes apoptosis through inhibiting ERK1/2 phosphorylation in epilepsy. Artificial Cells, Nanomedicine, and Biotechnology. 2020;**48**(1):298-304. DOI: 10.1080/21691401.2019.1671428

[67] Xu D, Robinson AP, Ishii T, Duncan DS, Alden TD, Goings GE, et al. Peripherally derived T regulatory and γδ T cells have opposing roles in the pathogenesis of intractable pediatric epilepsy. The Journal of Experimental Medicine. 2018;**215**(4):1169-1186. DOI: 10.1084/jem.20171285. Epub 2018 Feb 27

[68] Luo Y, Hu Q, Zhang Q, Hong S, Tang X, Cheng L, et al. Alterations in hippocampal myelin and oligodendrocyte precursor cells during epileptogenesis. Brain Research. 2015;**1627**:154-164. DOI: 10.1016/j.brainres.2015.09.027. Epub 2015 Oct 4

[69] Ma H, Lin H. Advances regarding Neuroinflammation biomarkers with noninvasive techniques in epilepsy. Behavioural Neurology. 2021;**2021**:7946252. DOI: 10.1155/2021/7946252

[70] Nutma E, Willison H, Martino G, Amor S. Neuroimmunology—The past, present and future. Clinical and Experimental Immunology. 2019;**197**(3):278-293. DOI: 10.1111/cei.13279. Epub 2019 Mar 11

[71] Abbott NJ, Friedman A. Overview and introduction: The blood-brain barrier in health and disease. Epilepsia. 2012;**53**(Suppl. 6):1-6. DOI: 10.1111/j.1528-1167.2012.03696.x

[72] Friedman A, Heinemann U. Role of blood-brain barrier dysfunction in Epileptogenesis. In: Noebels JL, Avoli M, Rogawski MA, Olsen RW, Delgado-Escueta AV, editors. Jasper's Basic Mechanisms of the Epilepsies [Internet]. 4th ed. Bethesda (MD): National Center for Biotechnology Information (US); 2012

[73] Baruah J, Vasudevan A, Köhling R. Vascular integrity and signaling determining brain development, network excitability, and Epileptogenesis. Frontiers in Physiology. 2020;**10**:1583. DOI: 10.3389/fphys.2019.01583

[74] Sukhovaia AI, Pimonov DA, Zabrodskaya YM. The inflammatory response in epileptic foci in pharmaco-resistant epilepsy. Russian Military Medical Academy Reports. 2020;**2**(S1):170-173. DOI: 10.17816/rmmar43420. (In Russ.)

[75] Sitovskaya DA, Litovchenko AV, Bazhanova ED, Skiteva EN, Zabrodskaya YM. Cytokine profile in the peripheral blood and the brain in patients with focal drug-resistant epilepsy. Sechenov Medical Journal. 2021;**12**(4):39-50. DOI: 10.47093/2218-7332.2021.12.4.39-50. (In Russ.)

[76] Litovchenko AV, Zabrodskaya YM, Sitovskaya DA, et al. Markers of Neuroinflammation and apoptosis in the temporal lobe of patients with drug-resistant epilepsy. Journal of Evolutionary Biochemistry and Physiology. 2021;**57**:1040-1049. DOI: 10.1134/S0022093021050069

[77] Rana A, Musto AE. The role of inflammation in the development of epilepsy. Journal of Neuroinflammation. 2018;**15**(1):144. DOI: 10.1186/s12974-018-1192-7

[78] Gaikova ON. Significance of cerebral white matter damage in pathogenesis of epilepsy. Bulletin of the Russian Military Medical Academy (Vestnik Rossiiskoi voenno-meditsinskoi akademii). 2002;**7**(1):35-42. (In Russ.)

Section 2

Medical Aspects of Epilepsy

Chapter 4

Psychogenic Non-Epileptic Seizures (PNES)

Nirmeen A. Kishk and Mai B. Nassar

Abstract

Psychogenic non-epileptic seizures (PNES) are a common presentation to the emergency rooms and neurology departments, and they are difficult to discriminate from epileptic seizures (ES). PNES present as paroxysmal time-limited, alterations in motor, sensory, autonomic, and/or cognitive signs and symptoms, but unlike epilepsy, PNES are not caused by ictal epileptiform activity. There is no exact known etiology or mechanism for PNES so far. The most recognized factors discussed in the literature include trauma and child adversity, dissociation, somatization, emotional processing, psychiatric comorbidities, coping styles, and family dysfunction. The use of a comprehensive assessment model may ease the transition of patient care from the diagnosing team to the outpatient treatment provider. Recognition of the characteristic clinical features of PNES and utilization of video-EEG to confirm the diagnosis are critical. Communicating the diagnosis, discontinuation of treatment for epilepsy (unless comorbid PNES and epilepsy are present), and implementing proper liaison with a multidisciplinary team with clinical psychologists, neurologists, and psychiatrists improve patient and healthcare outcome.

Keywords: PNES, DES, definition, etiopathology, management

1. Introduction

According to Hingray et al. [1], between 12 and 20% of adults presenting in epilepsy clinics have dissociative seizures.

Psychogenic non-epileptic seizures present as paroxysmal time-limited, alterations in motor, sensory, autonomic, and/or cognitive signs and symptoms that are not caused by ictal epileptiform activity, and positive evidence for psychogenic factors that may have caused the seizure is present [2].

PNES were formerly given different names including the name hystero-epilepsy, pseudo-seizures, and behavioral spells. However, most of these terms became abandoned in the literature because of being either vague or pejorative, implying that the seizures are unreal or fake. So, the accepted terminology in the medical community became psychogenic non-epileptic seizures (PNES), non-epileptic attack disorder (NEAD) [3], or dissociative non-epileptic seizures (DES) [4].

2. Epidemiology

The prevalence of PNES remains somewhat uncertain but has been estimated at up to 50/100000[3]; the incidence of video electroencephalography (vEEG)-confirmed PNES has been determined as 4/100000 per year [5]. However, data from epilepsy centers estimate a much higher incidence rate.

3. Etio-pathology

Up to now, there is no exact known etiology or mechanism for PNES. Some of the most commonly presumed factors include trauma and childhood adversity, dissociation, somatization, alexithymia and defective emotional processing, illness perception, family dysfunction, psychiatric comorbidities and personality factors, age, gender, and organicity (including comorbid epilepsy and anti-seizure medication use) [3, 6, 7].

4. Psychogenesis

Considering the previously mentioned factors, multiple theories for the psychogenesis or the mechanism by which PNES operate were hypothesized. All of these have agreed about the multifactorial nature of PNES that can be explained by different models.

One of the convenient proposed models for the psychogenesis of PNES is the one proposed by Bodde et al. [7]. This model shows five different layers or levels that highlight how each of these factors represents a heterogeneous group and may have a differential impact on the causation, development, and prolongation of PNES, emphasizing that not all factors have a similar impact. The proposed model is as follows:

Level 1. Psychological etiology

This includes the factors involved in the causation of PNES, such as sexual adversity or other traumatic experiences.

Level 2. Vulnerability

It refers to factors that act as predisposing elements for a person to develop psychosomatic symptoms like PNES, for example, personality factors, gender, neuropsychological impairments, organicity, and age. Many authors have pointed to the specific vulnerability of patients with PNES in terms of both their emotional "make-up" and their neuropsychological functioning.

Level 3. Shaping factors

Some factors can specifically shape the symptoms in the direction or form of "seizures" rather than other forms, for example, movement disorders or headache-like symptoms. A shaping factor may be a relative with epileptic seizures (symptom modeling) or the person himself having past history of epilepsy.

Level 4. Triggering factors

These are factors that create circumstances or situations that provoke and precipitate PNES, such as factors that refer to primary gain. Psychological mechanisms that transfer an emotional state into a seizure can be part of these triggering factors, such as dissociation and somatization. These factors explain why seizures occur on a

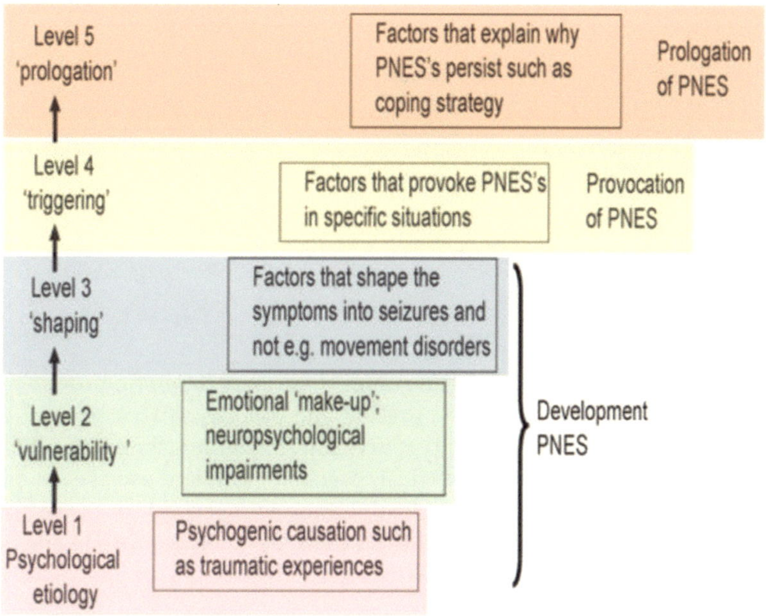

Figure 1.
Model of psychological factors involved in PNES [7].

specific day or in a cluster or why there is a period of remission. This differentiates PNES from conversion states that have a more predictable presentation.

Level 5. Prolongation factors

The previous factors are specifically important in the development of PNES, whereas prolongation factors are important in explaining why the seizures persist and PNES may become a chronic disorder. These factors tailor PNES frequency and resistance against therapy. Such modulating factors include the coping strategy of the patient and secondary gain aspects (**Figure 1**).

5. Predicting PNES: a multivariate approach

All the current research and studies aim to make that leap of "predicting" PNES, to change PNES from being a "diagnosis of exclusion" to being a "predictable," early detected diagnosis.

A multivariate approach may predict the development of PNES and provide useful markers for early identification of patients with potential PNES [6, 8, 9]. The multivariate approach proposed comprises the following:

5.1 The biopsychosocial/3P (BPS/PPP) psychiatric assessment

Multiple studies suggest that the biopsychosocial/3P (predisposing, precipitating, and perpetuating) model for approaching the diagnosis of PNES is one of the most comprehensive integrative models for screening and early identification of variables that can be readily and cost-effectively obtained in patients with non-diagnostic V-EEG evaluations, or eventually in an outpatient setting, and may prompt more rapid diagnosis and treatment [10–13]. See **Figure 2** [13].

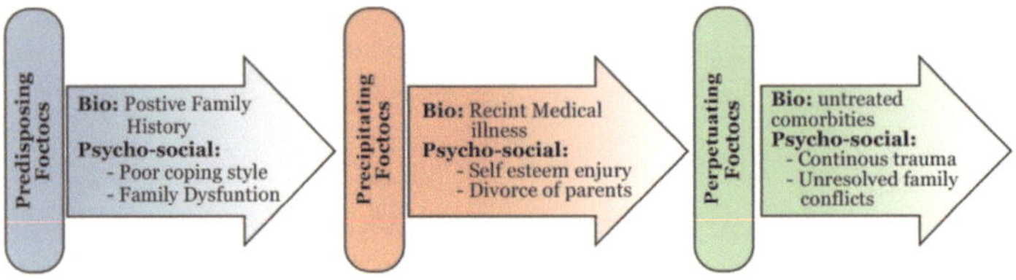

Figure 2.
Biopsychosocial conceptualization of PNES [13].

This involves a thorough psychiatric clinical interview to obtain precise history including demographic characteristics, present and past psychiatric history, medical history, family history, personal history, current living circumstances, and family dynamics to identify the possible biological, psychological, and social etiological factors that may interact as predisposing, precipitating (triggering), or perpetuating factors for PNES and present them in a BPS/3P (biopsychosocial/predisposing, precipitating, and perpetuating) formulation to establish a proper individualized treatment plan [10].

5.2 Clinical and neurophysiological assessment

Although none of the clinical signs by themselves carry a strong enough diagnostic value unless the psychiatric, neurologic, and neurophysiologic backgrounds are taken into account, the following clinical signs and serological and EEG findings were claimed to have a predictive value for PNES when integrated with the other previously mentioned psychological factors and semiological features [6, 8, 9, 11].

- *Self-reported length of the attacks:* Patients with PNES have longer (>2 minutes) events compared to patients with epileptic seizures, where the length of the attacks is usually less than or equal to 2 minutes [8].

- *Age of onset of seizures:* Patients with PNES have older age of onset compared to patients with epileptic seizures, with "30 yrs. old" as the average age of onset 12.

- *Frequency of seizures:* PNES have more frequent attacks than epilepsy; diagnosis entitles a frequency of at least 2 seizures per week [14].

- *Duration of illness (years since the first seizure):* Shorter duration/less years since the first seizures is considered a good predictor for PNES with an average of 8 yrs. since the first seizure [6, 8, 9].

- *Occurrence of an episode during clinic visits:* In a patient with "refractory epilepsy," the occurrence of an episode during clinic visits is a predictor of the episode being PNES with a high specificity (99%) and positive predictive value (PPV 77%) but a low sensitivity (3%) [12].

- *Prolonged PNES or NEPS:* Recurrent hospital admissions with prolonged PNES or NEPS (episode longer than 30 minutes) suggest PNES [6].
- *Response to medications:* Resistance to at least two anti-seizure medications is a predictor for PNES [14].
- *EEG findings:* At least 2 normal EEG studies are required to assume PNES15.

Added to that, the ILAE reported that predictors of PNES include the "rule of 2s" with an 85% PPV for PNES15. The rule of 2 s suggests that the diagnosis of PNES requires the following: at least two normal electroencephalography (EEG) studies with at least two seizures per week and resistance to two anti-seizure medications [6].

6. Patients' characteristics

In an attempt to discriminate factors underlying this heterogeneity and detect important predictors of dissociative seizures, Hingray et al. [1] identified dissociative seizure patients into three profiles; each had some factors in common, but from a statistical point of view, participants' trauma history pattern emerged as the strongest discriminating feature between these three profiles. Accordingly, Hingray et al. [1] named the identified patient subtypes according to their trauma history: Group 1, "No/Single Trauma"; Group 2, "Cumulative Lifetime Traumas"; and Group 3, "Childhood Traumas" (see **Table 1**).

7. Clinical presentation

i. *Semiology: Behavioral seizure manifestation:*

   According to Hingray et al. [1], cluster analysis data collected on patients with PNES were categorized using the proposed classification distinguishing five different semiological profiles, which were simplified to establish three groups based on categories most frequently used in the previous literature into hyperkinetic seizures (commonest semiology involves excessive movement of limbs, trunk, and head), paucikinetic seizures (seizures with stiffening and tremor), and syncope-like events or seizures (with atonia and loss of consciousness). The latter is less frequent [15].

ii. Phenomenology: *Subjective seizure experience*

   Many patients describe physical symptoms of panic or hyperventilation during their seizures without feeling anxious; it has been suggested that panic symptoms are more common in adolescents with PNES than in adults. Even in the absence of panic symptoms, most patients experience their seizures as confusing and beyond their control. At the same time, patients with epilepsy are more likely to conceptualize their seizure as a hostile agent acting of its own volition [1].

iii. *Autonomic seizure manifestations:*

More than one-quarter of patients with PNES give a history of ictal incontinence of urine; fecal incontinence is also reported. Sinus tachycardia is common but is more gradual in onset, less marked, and less persistent postictally than in epileptic seizures [15].

8. Confirming the diagnosis: A staged approach

Conversation analysis of history taking (**Table 2**) [16] and characteristic semiological and clinical features (**Table 1** [1]) and **Table 2** [16]) may help discriminate PNES from ES, but individually, they cannot not be a reliable diagnostic discriminator [17] (**Table 3**). To provide greater clarity about the process and certainty of the diagnosis of PNES and improve the care for the patients, the ILAE proposed a staged approach to confirm the diagnosis of PNES in which levels of diagnostic certainty were developed (see **Table 4**).

Key: + means history characteristics consistent with PNES, *PNES = psychogenic non-epileptic seizures, EEG = electroencephalogram.

9. Delivery of the diagnosis: communication protocol

The process of communicating the diagnosis is one of the most important and potentially effective therapeutic steps in the management pathway of patients with PNES with both immediate (within 24 hours of diagnosis presentation) and long-term

Criteria	Group 1 No/Single Trauma	Group 2 Cumulative Lifetime Traumas	Group 3 Childhood Traumas
Predominant gender	Male	Female	Female
Educational level	Low	High	Intermediate
Triggers	• Non-identifiable	• Identifiable	• Identifiable
	• Frustration more than anxiety	• Anxiety (80%) more than frustration (50%)	• Anxiety (84.1%) more than frustration (31.8%)
Trauma history	Non-significant	Significant Multiple emotional trauma (most common type)	• Significant
			• Childhood onset
			• Child sexual abuse and emotional trauma
PTSD Prevalence	Non-significant	PTSD in 33.3% of cases	PTSD in 63.6%
Comorbid epilepsy	43.4% (common)	16.7% (rare)	52.4% (commonest)
Seizures semiology	Non-hyperkinetic Seizures (paucikinetic 42.2%)	Hyperkinetic most common	Hyperkinetic: Non-hyperkinetic 1:1

Table 1.
Patients' characteristics in groups [1].

Diagnostic, linguistic, and interactional features yielded by conversation analysis	
PNES	**ES**
Patients tend to focus on the situations in which seizures have occurred or the consequences of their seizures rather than subjective seizure symptoms.	**Patients readily focus on the subjective seizure symptoms.
Subjective seizure symptoms may be listed but are not described in detail.	**Subjective seizure symptoms are given in detailed accounts with extensive formulation efforts (including reformulations, re-starts, neologisms, and pauses).
When the doctor tries to direct the patient's attention to particularly memorable seizures (e.g., the first, last, or worst seizure), patients commonly show focusing resistance by not providing further information or by generalizing rapidly to the description of their events in general.	**When the doctor tries to direct the patient's attention to particularly memorable seizures (e.g., the first, last, or worst seizure), patients readily provide more information about their subjective seizure symptoms in these particular seizures.
Patients tend to catastrophize their seizure experiences.	Patients tend to normalize their seizure experiences when talking to a doctor.
Patients prefer metaphors depicting their seizures as a place or space they traveled through or to which they were confined.	Patients tend to describe their seizures as acting independently (and often as doing something to the patient).

***features that revealed statistically significant differences between PNES and ES patients.*

Table 2.
Conversation analysis diagnostic features in PNES and ES [16].

Signs that favor PNES	**Evidence from primary studies**
Long duration	Good
Fluctuating course	Good
Asynchronous movements	Good*
Pelvic thrusting	Good*
Side-to-side head or body movement	Good**
Closed eyes	Good
Ictal crying	Good
Memory recall	Good
Signs that favor ES	Evidence from primary studies
Occurrence from EEG-confirmed sleep	Good
Postictal confusion	Good
Stertorous breathing	Good
Other signs	Evidence from primary studies
Gradual onset	Insufficient
Nonstereotyped events	Insufficient
Flailing or thrashing movements	Insufficient
Opisthotonus "Arc de cercle"	Insufficient

Signs that favor PNES	Evidence from primary studies
Tongue biting	Insufficient
Urinary incontinence	Insufficient
**Frontal lobe partial seizures excluded. **Convulsive events only.*	

Table 3.
Summary of evidence that supports the signs used to distinguish PNES from ES [6].

Diagnostic level	History	Witnessed event	EEG
Possible	+	By witness or self-report or self-description	No epileptiform activity in routine or sleep-deprived interictal EEG
Probable	+	By clinicians who reviewed recording or in person, showing semiology typical of PNES	No epileptiform activity in routine or sleep-deprived interictal EEG
Clinically established	+	By clinician experienced in diagnosis of seizure disorders (on video or in person), showing semiology typical of PNES while not on EEG	No epileptiform activity in routine or ambulatory ictal EEG during a typical ictus/event in which the semiology would make ictal epileptiform EEG activity expectable during equivalent epileptic seizures
Documented	+	By clinician experienced in diagnosis of seizure showing semiology typical of PNES while on video EEG	No epileptiform activity immediately before, during, or after ictus captured on ictal video EEG with typical PNES semiology

Table 4.
Proposed diagnostic levels of certainty for PNES [6].

reduction of PNES [18]. The summary of four reasonably detailed communication strategies that have been published [19–22] is shown in **Table 5** [23].

10. Treatment of PNES

I. Treatment of the underlying etiological factors and comorbidities:

Recognition and treatment of the “3Ps” (predisposing, precipitating, and perpetuating factors) are almost always necessary for symptom resolution. It may even be sufficient to treat the comorbid condition in conjunction with proper presentation of the diagnosis [12, 13].

II. Patient engagement:

Brief *psychoeducation* of the patient and *motivational interviewing* after presenting diagnosis can reduce ambivalence about treatment and facilitate behavioral change in favor of the patient’s health and give the patient a sense of control (internal locus of control) [20]. *Motivational interviewing* can be particularly useful in patients who find it difficult to trust their claimed diagnosis and thus recurrently seek new healthcare providers despite previous findings documenting PNES [24].

Covered topic	Communication points delivered to patient
Negative diagnosis	What you do not have (i.e., epilepsy) What you do not need (i.e., treatment with AEDs*) – unless needed for other indications
Diagnostic method	How diagnosis was made (i.e., video-EEG* captured typical event) "It is common!," frequently seen in long-term monitoring units
Genuine symptoms	Symptoms are real, not fabricated
Explanatory model (positive diagnosis)	Role of accumulating risk factors over time and automatic functional brain patterns
Suggestion	Some patients improve with reassurance that their events are not epileptic and once diagnosis is explained
Treatment and expectations	There are effective treatments Psychotherapy works though skills learning, "brain re-training" There is no sudden cure; treatment requires time and training

**AEDs = antiepileptic drugs, EEG = electroencephalogram.*

Table 5.
Diagnosis delivery: Summary of communication protocol [23].

III. Psychotherapeutic interventions:

A. *Cognitive behavioral therapy*

In a randomized controlled trial that compared cognitive behavioral therapy (CBT) to standard medical care, individual CBT was evaluated with a significant reduction in monthly event frequency after 12 sessions [25]. The following concepts were addressed in the CBT sessions: (1) treatment engagement; (2) reinforcement of independence; (3) distraction, relaxation, and refocusing techniques when episode is imminent; (4) graded exposure to avoided situations; (5) cognitive restructuring; and (6) relapse prevention.

B. *Psychodynamic psychotherapy*

Psychodynamic psychotherapy has not been examined as frequently as CBT, but favorable results have been demonstrated in uncontrolled studies using individual and group formats [26, 27].

C. *Family therapy*

Family therapy may be indicated when family system dysfunction is present since it is a contributor to symptoms of depression and to a poorer quality of life in PNES [28].

D. *Mindfulness techniques*

Mindfulness techniques promote the challenging of experiential avoidance while delineating personal values. In a case series that utilized a mindfulness-based treatment protocol, event reduction was attained using mindfulness techniques [29].

IV. *Pharmacotherapy:*

A. The pharmacologic treatment of patients should begin with early tapering and discontinuation of the anti-epileptic drugs (AEDs).

B. In people with mixed epileptic seizures (ES) and PNES, reduce high doses of AEDs or polytherapy if possible.

C. Use psychopharmacologic agents to treat comorbidities.

Protocol of personalized psychological interventions in PNES

Triage: • Patient's thoughts on diagnosis and potential treatment (locus of control, attributions, and perceived responsibility for recovery) • Seizures occurrence and response to seizures (seizure description, frequency, hospital contact, and medications) • Onset factors (home, work, and life events in the months prior to onset) • Current circumstances (home, family, work, pastimes, and social support) • Past history (other illness, traumatic events, and long-term life history) Treatment: • Treatment approach was based on a psychological formulation developed with the patient. • The broad outline of the treatment covered the following: psychoeducation to patients and their families to develop an understanding of PNES* and awareness of triggers, both external and internal; considering the context that may both prevent and perpetuate attacks; and identifying the attack prodromal phase and how to take remedial action. • While the models used were integrative and varied according to the formulation, intervention was predominantly delivered in a CBT* framework; other approaches were used on a case-by-case basis (see below). • Session 1: assessment and formulation • Sessions 2–10: interventions are used according to treatment targets that emerge from formulation: 1. When social factors predominate in cause and maintenance: Family therapy Interpersonal therapy Social interventions 2. When internal thought processes/personal conscious behavior predominate in cause and maintenance: Cognitive behavioral therapy Behavioral management advice 3. When internal conflicts such as grief or reaction to past trauma predominate in cause and maintenance: Mindfulness and compassionate mind Acceptance and commitment therapy Counseling Focused analytic therapy Dialectical behavioral therapy 4. When physiological states, current health problems, or habitual reactions to these problems predominate in cause and maintenance: Psychological treatment for sleep dysregulation Cognitive assessment remediation Behavioral management advice

**CBT = cognitive behavioral therapy, PNES = psychogenic non-epileptic seizures.*

Table 6.
Protocol for psychological interventions in PNES.

In an attempt to reach a consensus on a specific protocol of psychological interventions when dealing with PNES, Duncan et al. [30] proposed a protocol (see **Table 6**).

11. Evidence-based guide for management of PNES

The ILAE proposed the following management algorithm shown in **Table 6** [6] in an attempt to provide an evidence-based protocol for the management of PNES (**Table 7**).

Treatment steps	Direct evidence	Indirect evidence
Diagnosis Consider early Investigate (vEEG)	X X	
Assessment Characterize: Neurologic comorbidity Psychiatric comorbidity Social/family conflict	X X X	
Communication of diagnosis Explain: What PNES are not What PNES are	X	X X
Psychiatric/psychological treatment Patient engagement Psychotherapy: CBT for PNES Family therapy	X X X	X X X
Antidepressants	X	X
Case management		X
Rehabilitation		X

Note: vEEG = video electroencephalogram, CBT = cognitive behavioral therapy, PNES = psychogenic non-epileptic seizures.

Table 7.
Management of psychogenic non-epileptic seizure and evidence basis [6] (updated from [31]).

Author details

Nirmeen A. Kishk[1]* and Mai B. Nassar[2]

1 Department of Neurology, School of Medicine, Cairo University, Giza, Egypt

2 Department of Psychiatry, School of Medicine, Cairo University, Giza, Egypt

*Address all correspondence to: nirmeenkishk@kasralainy.edu.eg

References

[1] Hingray C et al. Heterogeneity of patients with functional/dissociative seizures: Three multidimensional profiles. Epilepsia. 2022;**00**:1-16

[2] LaFrance WC, Devinsky O. The treatment of nonepileptic seizures: Historical perspectives and future directions. Epilepsia. 2004; **45**(s2):15-21

[3] Brown RJ, Reuber M. Towards an integrative theory of psychogenic non-epileptic seizures (PNES). Clinical Psychology Review. 2016; **47**:55-70

[4] Goldstein LH et al. Cognitive behavioural therapy for adults with dissociative seizures (CODES): A pragmatic, multicentre, randomised controlled trial. The Lancet Psychiatry. 2020;**7**(6):491-505

[5] Rawlings GH, Reuber M. Health care practitioners' perceptions of psychogenic nonepileptic seizures: A systematic review of qualitative and quantitative studies, no. April 2018

[6] LaFrance WC Jr, Reuber M, Goldstein LH. Management of psychogenic nonepileptic seizures. Epilepsia. 2013;**54**(1):53-67. DOI: 10.1111/epi.12106. PMID: 23458467

[7] Bodde NM, Brooks JL, Baker GA, Boon PA, Hendriksen JG, Aldenkamp AP. Psychogenic non-epileptic seizures–diagnostic issues: a critical review. Clin Neurol Neurosurg. 2009;**111**(1):1-9. DOI: 10.1016/j.clineuro.2008.09.028. Epub 2008 Nov 18. PMID: 19019531

[8] Baroni G et al. Variables associated with co-existing epileptic and psychogenic nonepileptic seizures: A systematic review. Seizure. 2016;**37**:35-40

[9] Hill SW, Gale SD. Predicting psychogenic nonepileptic seizures with the personality assessment inventory and seizure variables. Epilepsy & Behavior. 2011;**22**(3):505-510

[10] Jimenez XF, Bautista JF, Tilahun BS, Fan Y, Ford PJ, Tesar GE. Epilepsy & behavior bridging a clinical gap in psychogenic nonepileptic seizures: Mental health provider preferences of biopsychosocial assessment approaches. Epilepsy & Behavior. 2016;**56**:149-152

[11] Elliott JO, Charyton C. Biopsychosocial predictors of psychogenic non-epileptic seizures. Epilepsy Research. 2014;**108**(9): 1543-1553

[12] Sahaya K, Dholakia SA, Sahota PK. Psychogenic non-epileptic seizures: A challenging entity. Journal of Clinical Neuroscience. 2011;**18**(12):1602-1607

[13] Stonnington CM, Barry JJ, Fisher RS. Conversion disorder. The American Journal of Psychiatry. 2006;**163**(9): 1510-1517

[14] Davis BJ. Predicting nonepileptic seizures utilizing seizure frequency, EEG, and response to medication. Eur Neurol. 2004;**51**(3):153-156. DOI: 10.1159/000077287. Epub 2004 Mar 12. PMID: 15017116

[15] Reuber M. Psychogenic nonepileptic seizures: Answers and questions. Epilepsy & Behavior. 2008;**12**(4):622-635

[16] Jenkins L, Cosgrove J, Chappell P, Kheder A, Sokhi D, Reuber M. Neurologists can identify diagnostic linguistic features during routine seizure clinic interactions: results of a one-day teaching intervention. Epilepsy & Behavior. 2016;**64**:257-261

[17] LaFrance WC, Baker GA, Duncan R, Goldstein LH, Reuber M. Minimum requirements for the diagnosis of psychogenic nonepileptic seizures: A staged approach: A report from the International League Against Epilepsy Nonepileptic Seizures Task Force. Epilepsia. 2013;**54**(11):2005-2018

[18] McKenzie P, Oto M, Russell A, Pelosi A, Duncan R. Early outcomes and predictors in 260 patients with psychogenic nonepileptic attacks. Neurology. 2010;**74**(1):64-69

[19] Hall-Patch L et al. Acceptability and effectiveness of a strategy for the communication of the diagnosis of psychogenic nonepileptic seizures. Epilepsia. 2010;**51**(1):70-78

[20] Duncan R. Psychogenic nonepileptic seizures: Diagnosis and initial management. Expert Review of Neurotherapeutics. 2010;**10**(12): 1803-1809

[21] Mellers JDC. The approach to patients with 'non-epileptic seizures'. Postgraduate Medical Journal. 2005; **81**(958):498-504

[22] Shen W, Bowman ES, Markand ON. Presenting the diagnosis of pseudoseizure. Neurology. 1990;**40**(5): 756

[23] Baslet G, Seshadri A, Bermeo-Ovalle A, Willment K, Myers L. Psychogenic non-epileptic seizures: An updated primer. Psychosomatics. 2016;**57**(1):1-17

[24] Lundahl B et al. Motivational interviewing in medical care settings: A systematic review and meta-analysis of randomized controlled trials. Patient Education and Counseling. 2013;**93**(2): 157-168

[25] Goldstein LH et al. Cognitive-behavioral therapy for psychogenic nonepileptic seizures: A pilot RCT. Neurology. 2010;**74**(24):1986-1994

[26] Barry JJ, Wittenberg D, Bullock KD, Michaels JB, Classen CC, Fisher RS. Group therapy for patients with psychogenic nonepileptic seizures: A pilot study. Epilepsy & Behavior. 2008; **13**(4):624-629

[27] Mayor R, Howlett S, Grünewald R, Reuber M. Long-term outcome of brief augmented psychodynamic interpersonal therapy for psychogenic nonepileptic seizures: Seizure control and health care utilization. Epilepsia. 2010;**51**(7):1169-1176

[28] Salmon P, Al-Marzooqi SM, Baker G, Reilly J. Childhood family dysfunction and associated abuse in patients with nonepileptic seizures. Psychosomatic Medicine. 2003;**65**(4):695-700

[29] Baslet G, Dworetzky B, Perez DL, Oser M. Treatment of psychogenic nonepileptic seizures. Clinical EEG and Neuroscience. 2015;**46**(1):54-64

[30] Duncan R, Anderson J, Cullen B, Meldrum S. Predictors of 6-month and 3-year outcomes after psychological intervention for psychogenic non epileptic seizures. Seizure. 2016;**36**:22-26

[31] Reuber M, House AO. Treating patients with psychogenic non-epileptic seizures. Current Opinion in Neurology. 2002;**15**(2):207-211

Chapter 5

Emerging Trends in the Management of Cryptogenic Epilepsy

Joyce Shuk Wan Chow and Tak Lap Poon

Abstract

Cryptogenic epilepsy, accounting for ~40% of adult-onset epilepsies and a lesser proportion in paediatrics, is defined as epilepsy of presumed symptomatic nature in which the cause has not been identified. It has a higher prevalence of refractory seizures when compared to those with idiopathic epilepsy (40 vs. 26%). These patients are usually treated with multiple anti-epileptic drugs, yet the total number of which used is inversely proportional to their efficacy. Moreover, these children may have significantly worse behavioural problems and can result in substantial cognitive impairments when older. Luckily, the number of cryptogenic epilepsy cases is diminishing due to better diagnostic abilities in recent years. We aim to divide this chapter into three parts. First, we hope to discuss our working algorithm and explain the use and advantages of different imaging modalities including high-field 3-Tesla MRI with morphological analysis for accurate localisation of the epileptogenic foci. We shall then elaborate the concept of the epileptogenic circuit and explore the selection criteria for more invasive approaches, such as depth electrodes and SEEG. Last but not the least, we aim to discuss the surgical treatments, including VNS and DBS, and their outcomes in these patients.

Keywords: cryptogenic epilepsy, MRI-negative epilepsy, invasive monitoring, SEEG, MEG, TMS, FUS

1. Introduction

Cryptogenic epilepsies account for ~ 40% of adult-onset epilepsies and a lesser proportion in the paediatric age group. The majority of the cause is not identified, but it has a higher prevalence of refractory seizures and a worse surgical outcome. This group of patients also present with diagnostic difficulties as there are no abnormalities found in the magnetic resonance imaging (MRI) of these patients most of the time. Yet, the seizure frequency cannot be reduced by medications, and the prolonged use of anticonvulsants also poses detrimental long-term neuro-cognitive effects, particularly in children.

The pre-surgical evaluation is a crucial step in the identification of possible epileptogenic foci in these patients. An exhaustive list of investigations, for example

3T MRI, positron emission tomography (PET), single-photon emission computed tomography (SPECT), magnetoencephalography (MEG) and even invasive electrode monitoring, may be indicated for suitable candidates. The pros and cons of each of these investigations may vary, but they may provide the essential clues for the underlying disease region. Treatment methods may vary widely due to the concordance of the results, laterality of the language area and the resectability of these lesions. Despite surgical advances, genetics in epilepsies may also shed light on the treatment of idiopathic epilepsies in the future.

2. Cryptogenic epilepsy

2.1 Definition and causes

The aetiological causes of epilepsy are typically classified by the seizure type or syndrome. However, aetiology is also an important and major determining factor in the treatment, prognosis and clinical course of the disease. In the recent report by the International League Against Epilepsy (ILAE), the aetiology can be divided into three main categories, namely genetic, structural/metabolic and unknown causes. Shorvon et al. [1] have further divided them into four distinct categories:

1. Idiopathic epilepsy
2. Symptomatic epilepsy
3. Provoked epilepsy
4. Cryptogenic epilepsy

Cryptogenic epilepsy is defined as epilepsy of presumed symptomatic nature in which the cause has not been identified. The key difference between idiopathic and cryptogenic epilepsy is that idiopathic epilepsy is an inherited type with predominantly genetic or presumed genetic origin.

2.2 Epidemiology

It is difficult to tell the exact number of cryptogenic epilepsies due to problems with assigning causation in usual practice. For example, the distinction between idiopathic and cryptogenic epilepsies is often blurred and can be arbitrary, and the cause can be multifactorial in some patients. However, cryptogenic epilepsy is still one of the most common causes in adult-onset cases, accounting for approximately 40% of the total cases [1]. In another population-based study done in the 80s in the US, the annual age-adjusted incidence per 100,000 population was 17.2 for cryptogenic epilepsies [2].

2.3 Prognosis

In general, most epilepsy cases can be treated with anti-epileptic drugs. The remission rates are as high as 80, and 50% of patients are able to continue a life without seizures after treatment discontinuation [3, 4]. However, cryptogenic epilepsies tend to have uncertain or poor prognosis in which seizures tend to recur despite exhaustive treatments. The risk of relapse in 2 years for idiopathic/cryptogenic seizure with an abnormal electroencephalogram (EEG) is 48% [5, 6].

These patients are often on multiple anti-epileptic drugs (AEDs) for a long period of time. The adverse effects of individual AEDs vary from fatigue, dizziness, mental slowness and skin reactions to haematological disturbances. Some patients may develop intolerability to AEDs and have to discontinue treatment early, yet the majority of patients will continue to be exposed to the AEDs for the rest of their lives. The prolonged use of AEDs may result in neurological symptoms of ataxia, dysarthria, tremors and deranged liver function [7]. Irritability and hostility are often seen with levetiracetam [8]. In the paediatric population, behavioural side effects combined with mental slowness may significantly affect the child's attention and schooling performance in the long run. Moreover, growth may also be stunted as suggested by some authors who found low serum calcium levels in children taking long-term valproic acid [9]. Hence, surgical treatment methods can be an alternative in the patients with refractive epilepsies for seizure control and to reduce the exposure to AEDs in the future.

3. Pre-surgical investigation

3.1 Clinical characteristic

To start the journey of pre-surgical workup for consideration of possible epilepsy surgery for drug-resistant epilepsy (DRE), a detailed interview with patient, patient's family and careers who can provide detailed witness history and past background is mandatory. A constructive interview includes a detailed description of patient's types of semiology during seizure attacks, recapitulation of all relevant past history, possible risk factors or aetiological factors. All possible epilepsy surgery cases are advised to be evaluated by a multi-disciplinary team conference according to the neuro-imaging, electrophysiological, neuropsychological and psychiatric findings based on the concept of 'six cortical zones' (**Figure 1**) [10]. This concept is based on the findings of all the pre-surgical evaluation tools and postulates the different zoning around the lesion identified. The goal of epilepsy surgery is to have maximal resection of epileptogenic zone but to have no or minimal surgical disruption of the surrounding eloquent cortex that may lead to permanent postoperative neurological deficit.

Temporal lobe epilepsy (TLE) is the most frequent syndrome in DRE. It accounts for ~40% of all patients with partial seizures and 15–20% of all types of epilepsy. Hippocampal sclerosis accounts for 60–70% of all TLE cases, while other structural aetiologies, including focal cortical dysplasia, tumours, vascular lesions, trauma, etc., happen in 10–15%. Remaining 15–20% patients are classified as Cryptogenic TLE. A study from Korea tries to elucidate the clinical phenotypes related to the prognosis. Good drug response group showed clinical characteristic including older age of onset, less initial precipitating events including febrile seizures, central nervous system infection, head trauma, less aura and automatism, less generalization of seizure and less EEG abnormality [11]. Such correlation of older age of onset of seizure with better seizure control prognosis was observed also in Italy group [12].

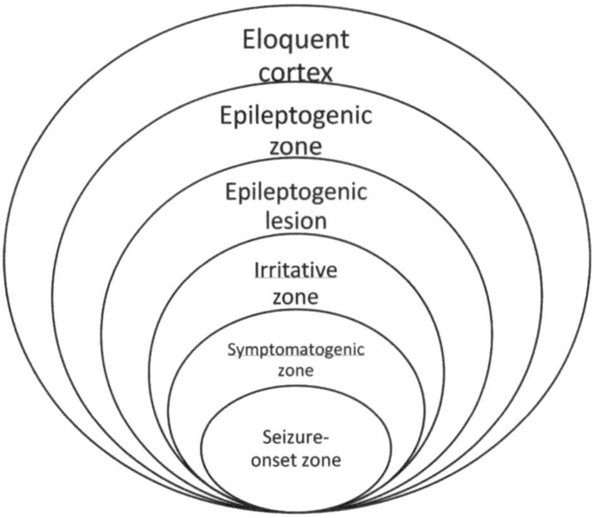

Figure 1.
Six cortical zones.

3.2 Neuro-imaging

About 20–40% of adult DRE patients can be classified as MRI negative or non-lesional or cryptogenic epilepsy. While no single investigation modality can provide optimal localization of epileptogenic foci in all cases, the use of multimodal imaging with a combined analysis of the findings of MRI, interictal PET and ictal SPECT can maximize the detection of the culprit [13, 14].

MRI scan of the brain constitutes the foundation of the imaging modalities. The recommended MRI epilepsy protocol in our hospital, the Queen Elizabeth Hospital, includes the following:

1. Volume acquisition T1W sequence acquired in oblique coronal orientation, orthogonal to long axis of hippocampus, covers whole brain in 0.9–1 mm partition

2. Oblique coronal T2WTSE and T2W FLAIR sequences orientated perpendicular to long axis of hippocampus, 2–3 mm slice thickness

3. Axial T2W or T2W FLAIR sequence of 3 mm slice thickness of whole brain

3T MRI system has better signal-to-noise ratio, spatial and tissue contrast resolution than 1.5T system and, therefore, it should be the gold standard of choice of MRI system for the epilepsy cases, together with Diffuse Tensor Imaging (DTI) and functional MRI functions [15]. The previous so-called 'cryptogenic epilepsy' cases by 1.5T MRI system turned out to be lesional cases after being rescanned by 3T MRI system with multichannel phased-array coils (**Figure 2**). Some centres are now using a 7T MRI system to confirm the suspicion in 3T MRI and locate any subtle lesions [16–18]. Apart from the increased signal-to-noise ratio, post-processing of MRI images by the application of voxel-based morphometric analysis

DOI: http://dx.doi.org/10.5772/intechopen.106382

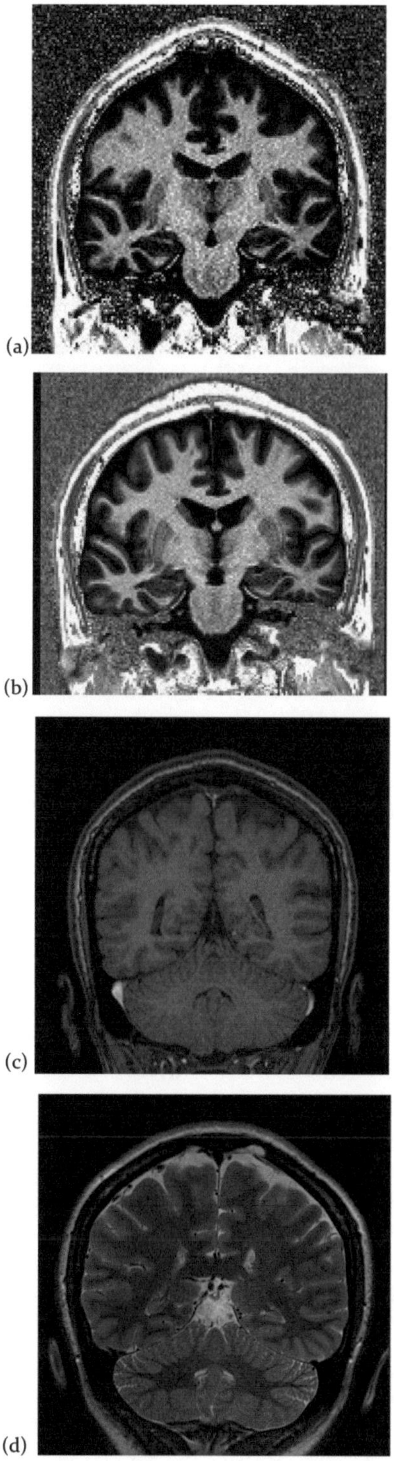

Figure 2.
A patient was regarded to be non-lesional epilepsy initially in 1.5T MRI (a); found to have cortical dysplasia in left temporal stem in 3T MRI (b); another epilepsy patient had very subtle lesion in right subependymal region in 1.5T MRI (c); and confirmed to be subependymal heterotropia by 3T MRI (d).

using morphometric analysis program (MAP) is another emerging direction to detect those subtle epileptogenic foci [13, 19, 20]. Wang et al. reviewed the use in 78 patients. About 56% had positive MAP, and complete surgical resection of MAP-positive regions was positively associated with good seizure outcomes. MAP-positive group rates were observed in 45% of TLE patients and 63% of extra-TLE patients [21].

FDG-PET (fluorodeoxyglucose positron emission tomography) scan is routinely used in pre-surgical evaluation. It is particularly helpful in cryptogenic TLE cases, as many of them displayed unilateral temporal hypometabolism in PET imagings. The predictive value of good surgical outcome is regarded up to 80%. In a retrospective review of 60 cases in China with unilateral TLE, one-third of all patients were cryptogenic groups with positive PET findings. There was no significant difference between surgical outcomes of lesion group and non-lesion group (Engel class I 68.3 and 68.4%, respectively) [22]. Similar study was carried out by LoPinto-Khoury et al. with 46 PET-positive cryptogenic TLE cases and 147 mesial temporal sclerosis cases. Engel class I rate did not differ significantly between two groups in two and five years (76% in 2 years and 75% in 5 years vs. 71% in 2 years and 78% in 5 years, respectively) [23]. Newer viewing platforms for PET scan including statistical parameter mapping (SPM) and three-dimensional stereotactic surface projection (3D-SSP) were employed to improve the sensitivities to detect epileptic foci in cryptogenic cases up to 60–70% [24].

With technological advancements, MRI scan images can be coregistered with FDG PET scan images and the MRI/PET scan. This further helps clinician to identify the subtle lesions in those previously believed cryptogenic epilepsy cases [25]. Toth et al. in Hungry had a prospective study of MRI/PET scan on 30 non-lesional and 30 lesional cases with discordant pre-surgical results. They concluded that the results of MRI/PET scan significantly altered the original plans in 19 of 60 cases [26]. In Hong Kong, this technology has been introduced since 2017 and we have more epilepsy patients that showed promising results in pre-surgical workup (**Figure 3**).

Ictal single photon emission computed tomography (SPECT) is used to provide information about regional cerebral perfusion, alteration of which is regarded to be hyper-activity and may be suggestive to be epileptogenic focus. Among those common substances used for ictal SPECT, 99mTc-bicisate (99mTc-ECD) had shorter injection latencies and a higher number of accurate ictal injections compared with 99mTc-hexamethyl propylene amine oxime (99mTc-HMPAO). It can correctly localize the epileptogenic focus in up to 97% of cases with known unilateral TLE and up to 90% in known or suspected extratemporal lobe epilepsy. For its application in cryptogenic epilepsy cases in order to improve the detection of epileptogenic foci, Yassin et al. proposed some innovative methods including subtraction ictal SPECT coregistered to MRI (SISCOM), statistical ictal SPECT coregistered to MRI (STATISCOM) and PET interictal subtracted ictal SPECT coregistered with MRI (PISCOM) [27].

Magnetoencephalography (MEG) helps to localize the epileptogenic zone and delineate the relationship between the suspected abnormality and the relevant regions in the brain. The placement of invasive electrodes can be guided by the MEG findings. A MEG-guided review of MRI may reveal subtle abnormalities and permit a precise surgical excision of the irritative zone. MEG is also indicated in patients with multiple intracerebral lesions, such as multiple cavernomas, in whom a sole epileptogenic lesion may be identified for lesionectomy [28]. In cryptogenic epilepsy

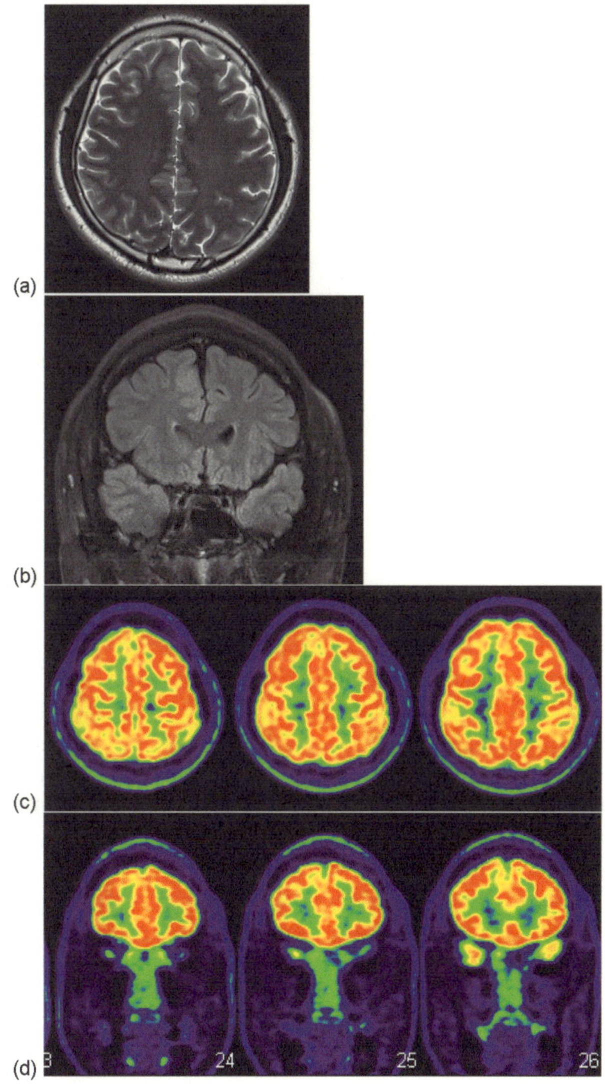

Figure 3.
A patient with frontal lobe epilepsy had negative 3T MRI finding (a) and (b); and subsequently, MRI/PET scan showed hypometabolism over left mesial frontal region (c) and (d).

cases, electric and magnetic source imaging (ESI/MSI) facilitate the prognostic assessment [29, 30].

3.3 Invasive intracranial electroencephalogram (EEG) studies

In general, the indications to consider invasive EEG monitoring are as the followings:

1. To define precisely the epileptogenic zone when non-invasive data are not concordant

2. To conclude the divergence of non-invasive data in different regions

3. To map eloquent cortical and subcortical function for respective surgery planning

4. To further validate the epileptogenic zone or provide information on prognostic value

5. To perform therapeutic treatment for active regions using thermocoagulation

Traditional invasive EEG modalities include subdural electrodes, intracerebral depth electrodes, epidural peg electrodes and foramen ovale electrodes. A comprehensive review on risks and benefits of using subdural and depth electrodes showed that the related complications include epidural or subdural haemorrhage, intracerebral haemorrhage or contusion, meningitis, oedema around the electrode, cerebral oedema, increased intracranial pressure, etc. The overall complication rate ranges from 0.4 to 6.6%.

Stereo-electroencephalography (SEEG) is gaining popularity to enable precise recordings from deep cortical areas in bilateral and multiple lobes without subjecting the patients to have bilateral large craniotomies. The key and most important concept in considering SEEG is to test individualised *anatomo-electro-clinical hypothesis*. Based on clinical history, semiology, preoperative imaging and vEEG data, the findings of SEEG help the clinicians to understand the spatial and temporal dynamics of seizures, that is where it starts, when and when it spreads. Study from the Italian group showed that SEEG is a useful and relatively safe tool to localize the epileptogenic zone with procedure-related morbidity of 5.6%. Other centres incorporate the neuro-robotic system in performing SEEG and showed comparable results. In general, SEEG had equivalent efficiency in determination of epileptogenic zone with lower operative morbidities and complications including CSF leak, intracranial haemorrhage and better tolerance to patients [31–34] (**Figure 4**). The application of SEEG in paediatric epilepsy patients was evaluated by Kim et al. Half of cryptogenic paediatric patients achieved postoperative seizure freedom [35].

Resective surgery in cryptogenic epilepsy cases usually can achieve Engel Class I seizure control in 30–60%. Invasive monitoring in terms of subdural grid, strip, depth electrodes and more advanced use of SEEG is a tool to attain a more precise localization of seizure. McGrath et al. in Yale have compared the surgical outcome of 48 cryptogenic epilepsy patients. Eleven patients underwent surgery without invasive monitoring, while 37 patients had invasive monitoring before their resective surgery or neuromodulative surgery. More patients with Engel Class I & II or III & IV outcomes underwent invasive monitoring (100 and 83%, respectively) [36].

4. Surgical treatment options

4.1 Multidisciplinary approach

As mentioned in the previous section, about 20–40% of adult DRE patients can be classified as MRI negative, non-lesional or cryptogenic epilepsy. Despite having more

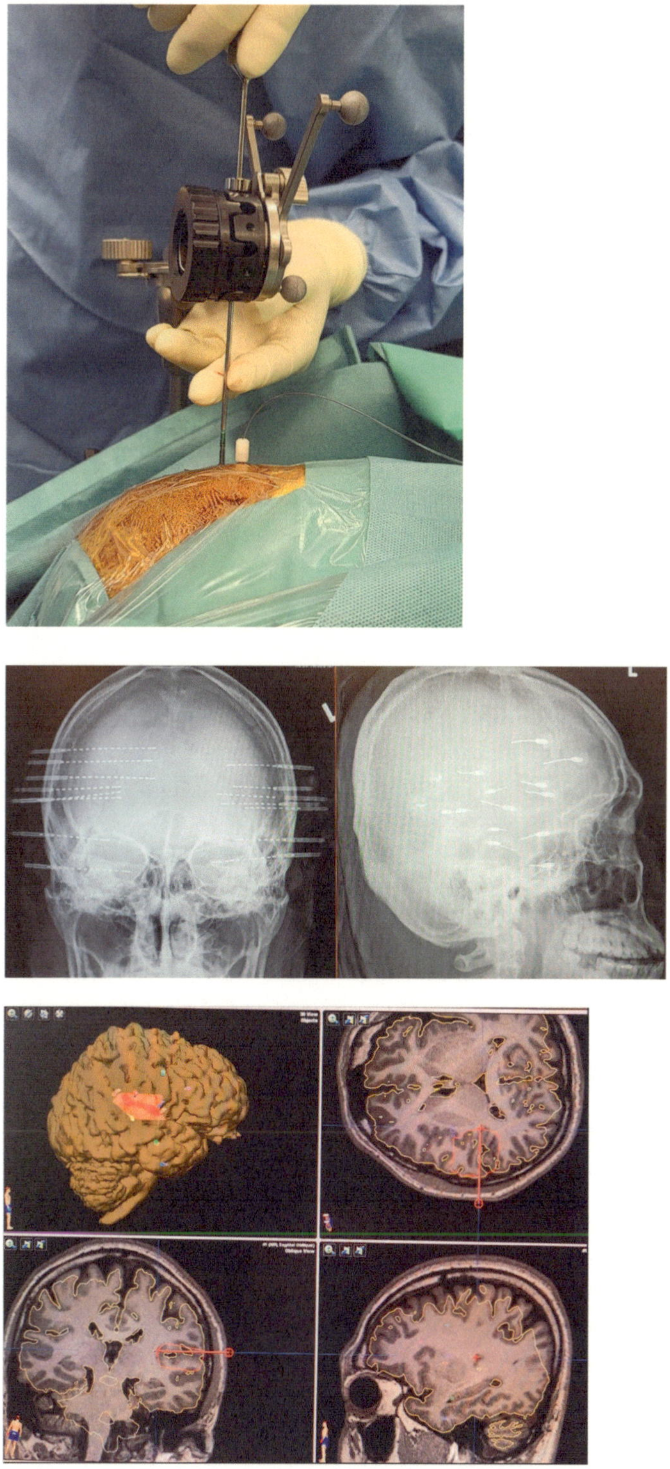

(a) (b) (c)

Figure 4.
Stereo-electroencephalography (SEEG) implantation in a patient with suspected right posterior temporal cryptogenic epilepsy (SEEG implantation) (a); post-implantation skull X-ray (b); and SEEG position coregistration with postulated epileptogenic zone in the neuro-navigation system (c).

advanced diagnostic methods in our armamentarium, the identification of the epileptogenic foci can still be an exercise of chasing the wind and clutching at shadows. The decision on how to treat these cryptogenic cases thus relies on a multidisciplinary approach to ensure the concordance of our findings.

In the usual practice, multidisciplinary epilepsy conferences are held regularly between neurosurgeons, neurologists, epileptologists, neuroradiologists and neuropsychologists to incorporate the different test results and opinions formulated for each case. Neuropsychologists are of particular importance in the evaluation of the baseline cognitive ability, lateralization of seizure focus and academic or occupational accommodations. This allows for a more tailored and holistic focus to assist the patient to return to work and normal life. However, some potential confounding factors may affect the test performance and its interpretation. For instance, patients on long-term AEDs may already have some cognitive side effects irrespective of the seizure semiology. Tasks that require memory may also be hindered, thus affecting the interpretation of laterality. Nevertheless, these results may be further dissected and correlated with the presenting symptoms in the conference meetings for the final decision management. We shall focus on the surgical approach in MRI-negative epilepsy patients in this chapter.

4.2 Resective surgery

Temporal lobe epilepsy (TLE) remains the most common cause of focal seizures in adults. Up to 30% of TLE cases can be non-lesional in MRI and requires complex pre-surgical workup. The surgical outcomes for non-lesional TLE patients are typically worse than lesional TLEs, with a pooled proportion of seizure-free patients 51 vs. 75% [37], and only 41–81% were documented to have Engel class 1 outcome at 1 year [38]. In TLE patients with concordant findings of the epileptogenic focus, anterior temporal lobectomy and selective amygdalohippocampectomy are indicated. Because these patients have no obvious lesion found in the temporal lobe and no hippocampal sclerosis, a formal neuropsychological evaluation, functional MRI +/- WADA test, is strongly encouraged to determine the language laterality and memory status prior to surgery. Invasive EEG monitoring can be an advantageous investigation, especially with dominant-side TLE patients, as the hippocampus may be spared if the invasive electrodes showed no activity during the ictus period.

Extra-temporal non-lesional epilepsy is even more difficult to visualize and resect completely. The outcomes of extratemporal non-lesional surgery are fair, with only 42% being seizure free at 2 years after surgery [39, 40]. Frontal lobes are the most common location for extra-temporal epilepsies; however, resection has a limited role in this group as it is not easy to identify the epileptogenic zone. Firstly, the interictal spikes may spread rapidly, making it difficult to even lateralize the lesion. Secondly, automatic clinical features may be due to a spread from other locations rather than a frank frontal seizure, as epileptogenic zones can be widespread. Lastly, the seizure focus may overlap with eloquent areas, such as the Broca's area and motor strip regions, which may limit the extent of resection. parieto-occipital lesions only account for ~ 1% of resections in some series.

In these cases, awake surgery may be indicated to help preserve function and excise the epileptogenic foci as much as possible. The use of intraoperative electrocorticography (ECOG) is another useful adjunct to ensure that the epileptogenic focus is completely resected (**Figures 5** and **6**). The region of abnormal

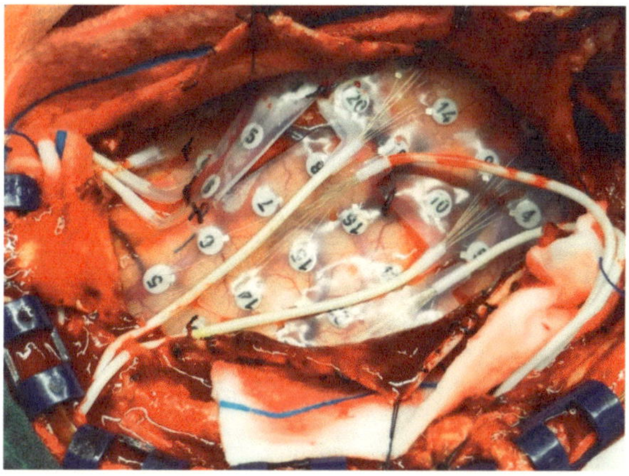

Figure 5.
Intraoperative photo of subdural grids used as electrocorticography. The epileptogenic foci were found to be in the area labelled '14, 15'.

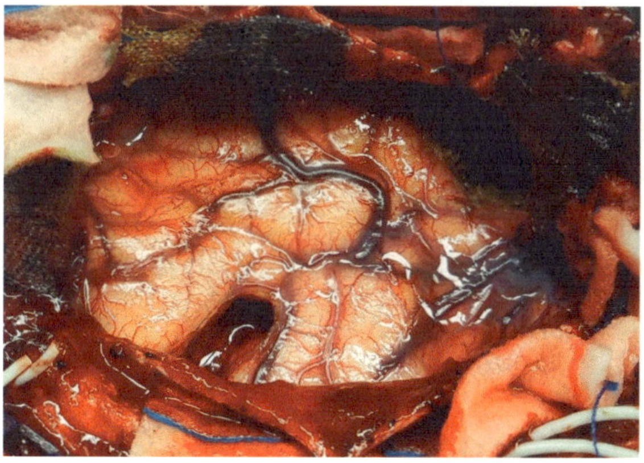

Figure 6.
Epileptogenic foci resected according to the labelled number '14, 15' on the grid with cavity seen.

electrical activity can be narrowed down using the labelled numbers prior to the procedure during the invasive monitoring period. The surgeon can then limit the zone of resection so as to avoid unnecessary neurological deficits, especially in lesions close to eloquent areas. Additionally, the ECOG enables the monitoring of inter-ictal spikes during the procedure, which is usually reduced after resection of the ictal zone.

Interestingly, the histopathological results were not entirely 'normal' in these patients. Focal cortical dysplasia (FCD) is the most commonly found pathology in MRI-negative epilepsy surgeries, with other aetiologies including gliosis, hippocampal neuronal loss or no pathology identified. In patients with non-concordant findings, resection is not recommended.

4.3 Neuromodulative surgery

Neuromodulative surgeries in terms of application of implanted devices and electrodes are regarded as palliative treatment for DRE cases that are not indicated for resective surgeries or disconnection surgeries. Vagus nerve stimulation (VNS) was approved by the U.S. Food and Drug Administration (FDA) in 1995, while the other two treatment modalities, Responsive neurostimulation (RNS) and Deep brain stimulation (DBS) of the anterior nucleus of the thalamus (ANT), had approval granted in 2014 and 2018, respectively [41]. Their mechanism of action and indications can be summarized as the followings (**Table 1**) [42, 43]:

	Mechanism of action	Indications
VNS	1. Alteration of noradrenergic projection system from the locus coerulus to connected regions including hippocampus, thalamus, hypothalamus, orbitofrontal cortex and cerebellum 2. Other involved possible circuitries including reticular activating system, central autonomic network and limbic system	1. Patients 4 years of age and older with focal onset seizures 2. Effective in individuals with primary generalized epilepsy
RNS	1. Only closed-loop system for epilepsy treatment 2. Stimulation of cortical neurons induces both immediate and long-term changes in local and distant sites involved in epileptic network	Patients 18 years of age or older with focal onset of seizures with less than two epileptogenic foci
DBS	1. Increased transmission of both excitatory and inhibitory neurotransmitters within basal ganglia-thalamocortical circuitry 2. Inhibition of action potential through sodium channel-mediated depolarization inhibition, direct distal axonal synaptic inhibition, depletion of neurotransmitters at distal terminals and potentiating the above mechanisms *via* direct stimulation	Patients 18 years of age or older with both focal or generalized onset of seizures

Table 1.
Possible mechanism of action and indications of VNS, RNS and DBS.

When we decide which neuromodulative surgical modality is most suitable for our patients, there are a few considering factors including the mechanism of action, device features, tolerability, patient preference and co-morbidities and disease focality. Concerning the long-term Outcomes, the number of studies showed no major differences in seizure control between different neuromodulative modalities with sustained improvement in quality of life [44–46]. In principle, VNS is effective for generalized-onset seizure. It has a diffuse effect and does not require localization. RNS depends on the localization of seizure-onset zones, which requires the analysis of invasive intracranial EEG recording results. DBS also does not require localization of seizure-onset zone, but seems it is more effective in patients with strong limbic system involvement. Besides, the safety profile of individual devices is another aspect to be considered (**Table 2**) [47–51].

In paediatric epilepsy patient group, VNS is traditionally believed to be the only choice of neuromodulative modalities. There is a recent review paper about the safety and efficacy of DBS in paediatric patients. Forty patients aged from 4 to 18 years old had received DBS treatment with targets including anterior nucleus of thalamus, centromedian nucleus of thalamus, hippocampus, subthalamic nucleus, hypothalamus and mammillothalamic tract. Overall, 12.5% of patients had achieved Engel class I seizure control, and 85% of patients had post-stimulation seizure reduction [52].

Devices	Safety profile
VNS	Possible stimulation-related adverse effects, for example hoarseness, cough and largyneal paresthesia. Worsening of obstructive sleep apnoea
RNS	Procedure-related primary burden. Possible adverse effects, for example haemorrhage, implant site pain or infection, headache and dysesthesia
DBS	Procedure-related primary burden. Possible adverse effects, for example implant site pain, paresthesia or infection, lead mistargeting, stimulating-related depression and memory impairment

Table 2.
Comparison of safety profiles of different neuromodulative surgeries.

In Hong Kong, VNS and DBS were available for our patients with DRE. First VNS was implanted in 1995. Since the government policy in funding subsidization in 2018, more cases were performed and totally, 70 devices were implanted. Half of them were adult patients and half of them were paediatric patients. DBS for refractory epilepsy cases were performed since 2015. Totally, 10 cases were performed by 2 epilepsy centres. In our hospital, Queen Elizabeth Hospital, we had four adult cases performed since 2020. The targets were all ANT *via* trans-ventricular route. There were no major perioperative surgical complications and neurological deficits, and there was no stimulation-related depression noticed. The mean seizure reduction rate >50% was ~60% at 3 months.

As mentioned, VNS, RNS and DBS have different mechanisms of action, preferred indications and their own unique adverse side effects, some centres borrow the concept of pharmacologic treatments with multiple anti-epileptic medications, and they had tried to consider polyneurostimulation in patient that had a suboptimal response to VNS treatment [53]. Mayo Clinic had a review on 131 patients who underwent neuromodulative surgeries from 1998 to 2021. Among those with VNS implanted, active dual stimulation occurred in 3 of 28 patients using RNS and 8 of 8 patients using DBS ($p = 0.006$). Patients who received VNS-DBS achieved a similar previous response to VNS ($p = 0.025$) and were unresponsive to more anti-epileptic drugs ($p = 0.02$). The VNS-RNS side had focal seizures more likely to have better electroclinical localization ($p = 0.005$), and more invasive intracranial EEG monitoring ($p = 0.026$) [54].

5. Emerging trends in cryptogenic epilepsies

5.1 Epilepsy genetics and future development

The modern era of technological advancement has pushed forward the progress of gene therapy. Since the completion of the Human Genome Project, more than 1800 disease genes have been identified. The first epilepsy-associated gene was discovered in 1995 in a family of autosomal dominant nocturnal focal lobe epilepsy (ADNFLE), the gene found was CHRNA4. In the recent decade, about 20 major genes were found to be associated with epilepsy, and they can be classified into different categories of voltage-gated, ligand-gated ion channels, subunits of acetylcholine receptors (CHRNA2, CHRNA4 and CHRNB2), subunits of sodium channels (SCN1a, SCN1B, SCN2A) and subunits of potassium channels (KCNQ2, KCNQ3), GABA (GABRA1, GABRA2).

Genetic disease accounts for approximately 70% of epileptic syndromes [55, 56]. In most circumstances, a syndromal diagnosis can be reached within the first few months of the disease in the infant onset epilepsies [57]. However, the diagnosis remains cryptogenic in about one-third of these patients despite clinical and EEG characteristics [57, 58]. In the routine clinical setting, testing of the autoantibodies, organic acids and neurotransmitters is used to find underlying autoimmune or metabolic causes for seizures. Genetic testing is the next step of investigation if the blood tests were negative. But the diagnostic yield is merely 10% in infantile epilepsies and 5% in epileptic developmental encephalopathies [56] using conventional methods. These methods may include genomic microarrays to detect DNA copy number variants (CNV), karyotyping for chromosomal abnormalities and single-nucleotide polymorphism (SNP) arrays to reveal regions of homozygosity. The reason for the low diagnostic yield is due to the fact that most epilepsies are actually associated with single-gene mutations instead. Traditional Sanger sequencing has been used by physicians to determine the nucleotide sequence of the exons of different genes; however, only one fragment of DNA can be run at a time. The cost is high when multiple genes are to be examined.

Next-generation sequencing (NGS) studies have provided a new light on the diagnosis of epilepsy genetics. There are three forms of NGS testing, epilepsy gene panel, whole exome sequencing (WES) and whole genome sequencing. The epilepsy gene panel can hold over 100–300 genes, which can detect molecular anomalies that could have been missed by traditional Sanger sequencing [59]. Whole exome sequencing (WES) allows simultaneous sequencing of exons of all the coding regions, that is ~1–2% of the whole genome, at a relatively low cost [55, 60], whereas whole genome sequencing (WGS) detects variants on the entire genome for both coding and non-coding regions. The diagnostic yield ranges from 20 to 50% depending on the different genetic panels that are available in the market and the clinical characteristics of patients [56, 61]. The cost of performing these tests was substantial in 2007 [62], but luckily the cost has been brought down to ~USD$1000 as NGS has been increasingly adopted into the routine clinical practice.

As the causes of early onset, infantile epileptic encephalopathies are heterogeneous and are often genetic, and NGS-based tests can be offered as a quicker method if an actionable condition is suspected. For instance, patients with cerebral creatine deficiency syndrome (SLC6AB, GAMT variant) can be treated with creatine replacement and phosphoglycerate dehydrogenase deficiency (PHGDH) with L-serine, or to manage with a ketogenic diet in glycine encephalopathy (GLDC) (**Table 3**). In patients with tuberous sclerosis, clinical trials have shown a reduction in seizures with the use of mTOR inhibitors [59, 65]. More clinical trials may be directed to the mTOR pathway in the future of targeted therapies in these patients. Potassium channel opener, retigabine, is a potential new drug indicated for KCNQ2-associated encephalopathy. This approach of precision medicine can tailor treatment methods for patients' needs and avoid detrimental side effects. Sodium channel blockers such as carbamazepine are the treatment of choice for SCN2A and SCN8A mutations, but they may cause worsening symptoms in Dravet syndrome (SCN1A gene mutation) [63].

Technical difficulties of NGS exist, a large amount of data retrieved need to be handled properly, and the complexity of the results requires a dedicated researcher for interpretation. Epilepsy has a large genetic heterogeneity, and a single epilepsy syndrome may be caused by 1 gene mutation in a family but can be due to many different genetic mutations in another. Moreover, additional studies have found new classes of gene mutations with poor geno-phenotypical relationships. Hence, it can be very challenging to determine the causative role of the detected gene mutation in NGS panels. Epilepsy in infants with migrating focal seizures (EIMFS) is pathologically due to the KCNT1 variant; however, this gene abnormality is also observed in many other epileptic syndromes. More than 20 different genes are also causatively linked to EIMFS in different studies [66, 67].

Gene variant	Target	Related syndromes	Treatment	Contraindications
1. Ion channelopathies and function-based therapies				
SCN1A	Sodium channel	Dravet syndrome, EIMFS, GEFS	N/A	Avoid sodium channel blockers [63] for example carbamazepine, oxcarbazepine, phenytoin
SCN8A	Sodium channel	DEE, familial myoclonic epilepsy, EIMFS	Carbamazepine, Oxcarbazepine, phenytoin	—
KCNQ2	Potassium channel	DEE, BFNE,	Retigabine	—
CACNA1A	Calcium channel	West syndrome, DEE	Ethosuximide, lamotrigine	—
GRIN2B	NMDA receptor	West syndrome, LGS, DEE	Memantine, radiprodil	—
CHRNA4	nAChR	NFLE	Transdermal nicotine	—
2. Metabolic diseases and substitutive therapies				
SLC2A1	Glucose transporter type 1	GLUT1 deficiency	Ketogenic diet	Phenobarbital, valproic acid, benzodiazepine [64]
GAMT	Guanidinoacetate methyltransferase	Cerebral creatine deficiency syndrome 2	Creatine replacement	—
POLG	DNA polymerase gamma	Mitochondrial disease	N/A	Valproic acid
3. Cell-signalling pathways and modification therapies				
NPRL	GATOR1 complex	FFEVF	Rapamycin and derivatives, e.g. everolimus, sirolimus	—
TSC1/2	TSC1/2	Tuberous sclerosis, focal dysplasia		—

BFNE, benign familial neonatal epilepsy; DES, developmental and epileptic encephalopathy; EIMFS, epilepsy in infancy with migrating focal seizures; FEEVF, familial focal epilepsy with variable foci; GEFS, generalized epilepsy with febrile seizures; LGS, Lennox-Gastaut syndrome; NFLE, nocturnal frontal lobe epilepsy; and nAhR, neuronal nicotinic acetylcholine receptors.

Table 3.
Genetic causes of epilepsy syndromes and treatment [56, 58].

Nevertheless, the ability to diagnose patients at an earlier age may prompt the development of specific drug therapies targeted to these mutated proteins in the future. The implications of NGS may also extend to potential therapeutic methods to prevent and avoid epilepsy development, and on-going studies are underway to limit epileptogenesis in tuberous sclerosis and Sturge-Weber syndromes [58, 68]. Other promising directions are towards the understanding of pharmacogenomics, gene therapy, and perhaps combining with artificial intelligence algorithms to predict pharmacoresistant patients [69].

5.2 Transcranial magnetic stimulation

Transcranial magnetic stimulation (TMS) is FDA approved for depression, migraines and obsessive-compulsive disorder (OCD). TMS is one of several newer treatments that can potentially offer epilepsy patients a tool for investigating the brain excitability, and a safe and non-invasive alternative to open traditional surgery. It allows probing the cortical excitability and analysing the excitatory and inhibitory brain mechanisms. TMS also had been used for the preoperative localization of the epileptogenic zone and mapping of eloquent area. Treatment for refractory epilepsy was another potential application [70]. Santiago-Rodriguez et al. in Mexico had conducted an open-label study for twelve epilepsy patients. Repetitive TMS (rTMS) was employed with 900 pulses, intensity of 120% motor resting threshold and 0.5 Hz frequency. Reduction of seizure frequency during the intervention period and follow-up period at 8 weeks were noticed but the differences were not statistically significant ($p = 0.19$) [71]. Application of low-frequency rTMS at 0.9 Hz with resting motor threshold stimulus intensity of 90% as treatment protocol was conducted also in Japan group, and they showed the frequency of all seizure types, complex partial seizures (CPSs) and simple partial seizures were reduced by 19.1, 35.9, and 7.4%. A trend of improvement, though not statistically significant, was demonstrated [72]. Lefaucheur et al. proposed guidelines established by a group of European experts on the therapeutic use of rTMS in other neurological disorders. In his paper, one sham-controlled low-frequency rTMS trial was quoted with seven patients with focal neocortical DRE received three treatment sessions with the following treatment plan: 10 sessions delivered by means of a figure-of-8-coil, a round coil, or a sham coil at 0.5 Hz and 90% of RMT over the cortical focus (1500 pulses/session). No difference in mean seizure rate was detected with one patient who had seizure rebound [73].

The other side of the coin in the use of TMS as potential treatment of refractory epilepsy is that there is a risk of TMS-triggered seizure attack. George and Belmaker mentioned patients with focal or generalized encephalopathy, severe head trauma, non-treated epilepsy, family history of epilepsy in first-degree relatives, heavy alcohol use, severe cardiac disease, increased intracranial pressure, medications that lower seizure threshold, etc., will have a relatively higher risk to have such seizure attack [74]. The general risk of seizures with TMS was ~0.08/1000.

Boston group done a review of over 70 articles related to the use of TMS-EMG and TMS-EEG in elucidating the mechanisms of action of anti-epileptic drugs (AEDs) and discovering potential new AEDs, and the use of rTMS in the treatment of seizures. For diagnostic potential, TMS-derived biomarkers can facilitate the measurement of AED target engagement and the study of pharmacokinetic and pharmacodynamic behaviours in order to predict the efficacy of different AED usage in epilepsy patients. For therapeutic potential, there is a trend to have favourable results [75]. Tsuboyama in the same group had another study to investigate the TMS-EMG metrics (**Table 4**) [76]. These findings imply that TMS may have a potential role in the optimization of AED regimens for epilepsy patients. Similar findings were reported by Bauer et al. also [77].

5.3 Focused USG

Neuromodulative surgeries in terms of DBS, VNS and RNS as treatment of refractory epilepsy cases were well established. Focused ultrasound (FUS) is considered as a non-invasive new armamentarium that can ablate the epileptogenic focus and modulate neuronal circuits or activities. The transducer in FUS is designed to transmit the acoustic energy only and directly to the chosen target according to the

TMS-EMG parameter	Purposed mechanism
Resting motor threshold (rMT)	Cortical motor neuron voltage-gated sodium channel-mediated membrane excitability
Cortical silent period (CSP)	$GABA_B$-mediated and $GABA_A$-mediated motor cortex inhibition
Short-interval intracortical inhibition (SICI)	$GABA_A$-mediated regional cortical inhibition
Intracortical facilitation (ICF)	Glutamate (NMDA and AMAPA receptor types)-mediated excitation
Long-interval intracortical inhibition (LICI)	$GABA_B$-mediated inhibition and (likely) $GABA_A$-mediated network inhibition

Table 4.
Transcranial magnetic stimulation-electromyography (TMS-EMG) metrics.

preoperative planning. Different intensity serves in different mechanisms of treatment. High-intensity FUS (~1000 W/cm^2) execute the thermoablation effect, while low-intensity mode (~3 W/cm^2) showed neuromodulatory effects and suppressive effects on the frequency of epileptic signal bursts. The proposed mechanism of action of low-intensity FUS included the following [78]:

1. Cavitation or eruption of ultrasound-induced gas bubbles causes changes in neural membrane

2. Increase of conductance of potassium channel in membrane and results in reduced resting action potential and increased firing

3. Excitation in mechanosensitive membrane induced by radiation force

Taipei Veterans General Hospital epilepsy surgery team employed a neuronavigation-guided low-intensity FUS system (ceiling spatial-peak temporal-average intensity level = 2.8 W/cm^3, duty cycle = 30%, modulating duration = 10 min) to deliver to the seizure onset zone localized by stereo-electroencephalography (SEEG) in six patients. A decrease in seizure frequency was observed in two patients within 3 days recording with significant changes in spectral power of SEEG at the targeted electrodes [79].

Regarding the safety in application of low-intensity FUS in the treatment of epilepsy, early in 2008, Tyler et al. have investigations with *ex vivo* preparations in mouse. They showed that repeated stimulation of hippocampus slices did not result in significant changes to cytoarchitecture or integrity and integrity of the blood-brain barrier was not disturbed [80]. Zou et al. in China also showed no significant brain tissue damage after low-intensity FUS application to acute epileptic Monkeys [81]. Concerning the application to human cases, Monteith et al. had tested the feasibility of using FUS for temporal lobe epilepsy by using cadaveric skulls [82]. Abe et al. in Japan reported the first case of transcranial magnetic resonance-guided FUS (MRgFUS) for mesial temporal lobe epilepsy [83]. Further study in UCLA group on eight temporal lobe epilepsy patients before and after treatment with FUS using intensities up to 5760 mW/cm showed that there was no detectable damage to the tissue in the histological analysis of the resected specimens, and the neuropsychological testing results showed no significant changes after the treatment [84].

Though there are promising results in treatment of refractory epilepsy, FUS is considered to have some limitations. One of them is the limitation of treatment target size. FUS cannot completely ablate an epileptogenic lesion larger than 1 cm^3 as convergence of ultrasound waves is required. Another challenge is the gantry of ultrasound waves with reference to the location of a target in skull base region. It may be difficult to achieve a high enough treatment efficiency to cause thermal ablation in mesial temporal structure including the hippocampus and amygdala for those mesial temporal lobe epilepsy cases [85].

6. Conclusions

Cryptogenic epilepsy remains a challenging entity and difficult disease to treat. The advanced imaging technologies and invasive monitoring methods help to localize the epileptogenic focus more accurately. Innovative methods of treatment may be an alternative method of treatment particularly in those lesions with high surgical risks.

Acknowledgements

The authors acknowledge Department of Neurosurgery, Queen Elizabeth Hospital, Hong Kong.

Conflict of interest

The authors declare no conflict of interest.

Author details

Joyce Shuk Wan Chow* and Tak Lap Poon
Queen Elizabeth Hospital, Hong Kong

*Address all correspondence to: csw814@ha.org.hk

References

[1] Shorvon SD. The etiologic classification of epilepsy. Epilepsia. 2011;**52**(6):1052-1057

[2] Zarrelli MM, Beghi E, Rocca WA, Hauser WA. Incidence of epileptic syndromes in Rochester, Minnesota: 1980-1984. Epilepsia. 1999;**40**(12):1708-1714

[3] Annegers JF, Hauser WA, Elveback LR. Remission of seizures and relapse in patients with epilepsy. Epilepsia. Dec. 1979;**20**(6):729-737

[4] Sillanpää M, Schmidt D. Natural history of treated childhood-onset epilepsy: Prospective, long-term population-based study. Brain. Mar. 2006;**129**(Pt 3):617-624

[5] Berg AT, Shinnar S. The risk of seizure recurrence following a first unprovoked seizure: A quantitative review. Neurology. Jul. 1991;**41**(7):965-972

[6] Beghi E. The epidemiology of epilepsy. Neuroepidemiology. 2020;**54**(2):185-191

[7] Nakazawa Y, Ohkawa T. Study of the side effects of long-term anticonvulsant treatment. Folia Psychiatrica et Neurologica Japonica. 1980;**34**(3):271-275

[8] Halma E, de Louw AJA, Klinkenberg S, Aldenkamp AP, IJff DM, Majoie M. Behavioral side-effects of levetiracetam in children with epilepsy: A systematic review. Seizure. Oct. 2014;**23**(9):685-691

[9] Lee H-S, Wang S-Y, Salter DM, Wang C-C, Chen S-J, Fan H-C. The impact of the use of antiepileptic drugs on the growth of children. BMC Pediatric. 2013;**13**(1):211

[10] Poon TL, Lui CHT, Chan I, Siu DYW. Updated review: Drug-resistant epilepsy and presurgical evaluation of epilepsy surgery. Hong Kong Medical Journal. 2018;**24**(6):610-616

[11] Kim J, Kim SH, Lim SC, Kim W, Shon YM. Clinical characteristics of patients with benign nonlesional temporal lobe epilepsy. Neuropsychiatric Disease and Treatment. 2016;**12**: 1887-1891

[12] Aguglia U et al. Age at onset predicts good seizure outcome in sporadic non-lesional and mesial temporal sclerosis based temporal lobe epilepsy. Journal of Neurology, Neurosurgery, and Psychiatry. 2011;**82**(5):555-560

[13] Wang S et al. Multimodal noninvasive evaluation in MRI-negative operculoinsular epilepsy. Journal of Neurosurgery. 2020;**132**(5):1334-1344

[14] Juhász C, John F. Utility of MRI, PET, and ictal SPECT in presurgical evaluation of non-lesional pediatric epilepsy. Seizure. 2020;**77**:15-28

[15] Degnan AJ, Samtani R, Paudel K, Levy LM. Neuroimaging of epilepsy: A review of MRI findings in uncommon etiologies and atypical presentations of seizures. Future Neurology. 2014;**9**(4):431-448

[16] Feldman RE, Delman BN, Dyvorne H, Rutland JW, Yoo J. 7T study of patients with previously normal MRI exams. Plos One. 2019;**14**(3):1-24

[17] Sone D. Making the invisible visible: Advanced neuroimaging techniques in focal epilepsy. Frontiers in Neuroscience. 2021;**15**:1-10

[18] Chen C et al. 7T MRI with post-processing for the presurgical evaluation of pharmacoresistant focal epilepsy. Therapeutic Advances in Neurological Disorders. 2021;**14**:1-14

[19] Wang ZI et al. Linking MRI postprocessing with magnetic source imaging in MRI-negative epilepsy. Annals of Neurology. 2014;**75**(5):759-770

[20] Delev D et al. A multimodal concept for invasive diagnostics and surgery based on neuronavigated voxel-based morphometric MRI postprocessing data in previously nonlesional epilepsy. Journal of Neurosurgery. 2018;**128**(4):1178-1186

[21] Wang W et al. Voxel-based morphometric magnetic resonance imaging postprocessing in non-lesional pediatric epilepsy patients using pediatric normal databases. European Journal of Neurology. 2019;**26**(7):969-e71

[22] Feng R et al. Surgical treatment of MRI-negative temporal lobe epilepsy based on PET: A retrospective cohort study. Stereotactic and Functional Neurosurgery. 2014;**92**(6):354-359

[23] LoPinto-Khoury C, Sperling MR, Skidmore C, Nei M, Evans J, Sharan A, et al. Surgical outcome in PET-positive, MRI-negative patients with temporal lobe epilepsy. Epilepsia. 2012 Feb;**53**(2):342-348

[24] Zhou H et al. Localizing epileptic foci before surgery in patients with MRI-negative refractory epilepsy using statistical parameter mapping and three-dimensional stereotactic surface projection based on 18F-FDG PET. Frontiers in Bioengineering and Biotechnology. 2022;**9**:1-11

[25] Sun K et al. Voxel-based morphometric MRI post-processing and PET/MRI co-registration reveal subtle abnormalities in cingulate epilepsy. Epilepsy Research. 2021;**171**:106568

[26] Tóth M et al. The role of hybrid FDG-PET/MRI on decision-making in presurgical evaluation of drug-resistant epilepsy. BMC Neurology. 2021;**21**(1):1-20

[27] Yassin A et al. Use of innovative SPECT techniques in the presurgical evaluation of patients with nonlesional extratemporal drug-resistant epilepsy. Molecular Imaging. 2021;**2021**. [Online Article]

[28] Poon TL, Cheung FC, Lui CHT. Magnetoencephalography and its role in evaluation for epilepsy surgery. Hong Kong Medical Journal. 2010;**16**(1):44-47

[29] Mohamed IS et al. Utility of magnetic source imaging in nonlesional focal epilepsy: A prospective study. Neurosurgical Focus. 2020;**48**(4):1-11

[30] Ntolkeras G, Tamilia E, AlHilani M, Bolton J, Grant PE, Prabhu SP, et al. Presurgical accuracy of dipole clustering in MRI-negative pediatric patients with epilepsy: Validation against intracranial EEG and resection. Clinical Neurophysiology. 2021 Mar 26 [In press]

[31] González-Martínez J et al. Technique, results, and complications related to robot-assisted stereoelectroencephalography. Neurosurgery. 2016;**78**(2):169-179

[32] Cardinale F et al. A new tool for touch-free patient registration for robot-assisted intracranial surgery: Application accuracy from a phantom study and a retrospective surgical series. Neurosurgical Focus. 2017;**42**(5):1-7

[33] Wellmer J et al. Risks and benefits of invasive epilepsy surgery workup with

implanted subdural and depth electrodes. Epilepsia. 2012;**53**(8):1322-1332

[34] Kahane P, Landré E, Minotti L, Francione S, Ryvlin P. The Bancaud and Talairach view on the epileptogenic zone: A working hypothesis. Epileptic Disorders. 2006;**8**(SUPPL. 2):16-26

[35] Kim W et al. The role of stereo-electroencephalography to localize the epileptogenic zone in children with nonlesional brain magnetic resonance imaging. Epilepsy Research. 2022;**179**:106828

[36] McGrath H et al. Optimizing the surgical management of MRI-negative epilepsy in the neuromodulation era. Epilepsia Open. 2022;**7**(1):151-159

[37] Téllez-Zenteno JF, Hernández Ronquillo L, Moien-Afshari F, Wiebe S. Surgical outcomes in lesional and non-lesional epilepsy: A systematic review and meta-analysis. Epilepsy Research. May 2010;**89**(2-3):310-318

[38] Muhlhofer W, Tan YL, Mueller SG, Knowlton R. MRI-negative temporal lobe epilepsy—What do we know? Epilepsia. 2017;**58**(5):727-742

[39] See S-J, Jehi LE, Vadera S, Bulacio J, Najm I, Bingaman W. Surgical outcomes in patients with extratemporal epilepsy and subtle or normal magnetic resonance imaging findings. Neurosurgery. Jul. 2013;**73**(1):67-68

[40] So EL, Lee RW. Epilepsy surgery in MRI-negative epilepsies. Current Opinion in Neurology. 2014 Apr 1;**27**(2):206-212

[41] Ryvlin P, Jehi LE. Neuromodulation for refractory epilepsy. Epilepsy Current. 2022;**22**(1):11-17

[42] Markert MS, Fisher RS. Neuromodulation – Science and practice in epilepsy: Vagus nerve stimulation, thalamic deep brain stimulation, and responsive neurostimulation. Expert Review of Neurotherapeutics. 2019;**19**(1):17-29

[43] Ali I, Houck K. Neuromodulation in pediatric epilepsy. Neurologic Clinics. 2021;**39**(3):797-810

[44] Gooneratne IK et al. Comparing neurostimulation technologies in refractory focal-onset epilepsy. Journal of Neurology, Neurosurgery, and Psychiatry. 2016;**87**(11):1174-1182

[45] Boon P, De Cock E, Mertens A, Trinka E. Neurostimulation for drug-resistant epilepsy: A systematic review of clinical evidence for efficacy, safety, contraindications and predictors for response. Current Opinion in Neurology. 2018;**31**(2):198-210

[46] Schulze-Bonhage A. Long-term outcome in neurostimulation of epilepsy. Epilepsy & Behavior. 2019;**91**:25-29

[47] Nune G, DeGiorgio C, Heck C. Neuromodulation in the treatment of epilepsy. Current Treatment Options Neurology. 2015 Oct;**17**(10):1-6

[48] Dalkilic EB. Neuro stimulation devices used in treatment of epilepsy. Current Treatment Options in Neurology. 2017 Feb;**19**(2):1-7

[49] Benbadis SR et al. Putting it all together: Options for intractable epilepsy: An updated algorithm on the use of epilepsy surgery and neurostimulation. Epilepsy & Behavior. 2018;**88**:33-38

[50] Soltani BA, Sharan I, Sharan A. Neuromodulation and epilepsy. 2018. Available from: https://practical

neurology.com/articles/2018-oct/neuromodulation-and-epilepsy

[51] Wong S, Mani R, Danish S. Comparison and selection of current implantable anti-epileptic devices. Neurotherapeutics. 2019;**16**(2):369-380

[52] Yan H et al. A systematic review of deep brain stimulation for the treatment of drug-resistant epilepsy in childhood. Journal of Neurosurgery. Pediatrics. 2019;**23**(3):274-284

[53] Park HR et al. The role of anterior thalamic deep brain stimulation as an alternative therapy in patients with previously failed vagus nerve stimulation for refractory epilepsy. Stereotactic and Functional Neurosurgery. 2019;**97**(3):176-182

[54] Freund B, Grewal SS, Middlebrooks EH, Moniz-Garcia D, Feyissa AM, Tatum WO. Dual-device neuromodulation in epilepsy. World Neurosurgery. 2022;**161**:e596-e601

[55] Striano P, Minassian BA. From genetic testing to precision medicine in epilepsy. Neurotherapeutics. 2020;**17**(2):609-615

[56] Dunn P et al. Next generation sequencing methods for diagnosis of epilepsy syndromes. Frontiers in Genetics. 2018;**9**(Feb):1-11

[57] Sarisjulis N, Gamboni B, Plouin P, Kaminska A, Dulac O. Diagnosing idiopathic/cryptogenic epilepsy syndromes in infancy. Archives of Disease in Childhood. 2000;**82**(3):226-230

[58] Nabbout R, Kuchenbuch M. Impact of predictive, preventive and precision medicine strategies in epilepsy. Nature Reviews Neurology. 2020;**16**(12):674-688

[59] Myers KA, Johnstone DL, Dyment DA. Epilepsy genetics: Current knowledge, applications, and future directions. Clinical Genetics. 2019;**95**(1):95-111

[60] Hamdan FF et al. High rate of recurrent de novo mutations in developmental and epileptic encephalopathies. American Journal of Human Genetics. 2017;**101**(5):664-685

[61] Mercimek-Mahmutoglu S et al. Diagnostic yield of genetic testing in epileptic encephalopathy in childhood. Epilepsia. 2015;**56**(5):707-716

[62] Phillips KA et al. Methodological issues in assessing the economic value of next-generation sequencing tests: Many challenges and not enough solutions. Value in Health. 2018;**21**(9):1033-1042

[63] Wirrell EC, Nabbout R. Recent advances in the drug treatment of Dravet syndrome. CNS Drugs. 2019;**33**(9):867-881

[64] Klepper J, Voit T. Facilitated glucose transporter protein type 1 (GLUT1) deficiency syndrome: Impaired glucose transport into brain - A review. European Journal of Pediatrics. 2002;**161**(6):295-304

[65] Li M et al. Efficacy and safety of mTOR inhibitors (rapamycin and its analogues) for tuberous sclerosis complex: A meta-analysis. Orphanet Journal of Rare Diseases. 2019;**14**(1):39

[66] Lim CX, Ricos MG, Dibbens LM, Heron SE. KCNT1 mutations in seizure disorders: The phenotypic spectrum and functional effects. Journal of Medical Genetics. 2016;**53**(4):217-225

[67] Burgess R et al. The genetic landscape of epilepsy of infancy with migrating focal seizures. Annals of Neurology. 2019;**86**(6):821-831

[68] Jansen AC et al. Long-term, prospective study evaluating clinical and molecular biomarkers of epileptogenesis in a genetic model of epilepsy–tuberous sclerosis complex. Impact. 2019;**2019**(4):6-9

[69] An S et al. Predicting drug-resistant epilepsy—a machine learning approach based on administrative claims data. Epilepsy & Behavior. 2018;**89**:118-125

[70] Kimiskidis VK. Transcranial magnetic stimulation for drug-resistant epilepsies: Rationale and clinical experience. European Neurology. 2010;**63**(4):205-210

[71] Santiago-Rodríguez E, Cárdenas-Morales L, Harmony T, Fernández-Bouzas A, Porras-Kattz E, Hernández A. Repetitive transcranial magnetic stimulation decreases the number of seizures in patients with focal neocortical epilepsy. Seizure. 2008;**17**(8):677-683

[72] Kinoshita M, Ikeda A, Begum T, Yamamoto J, Hitomi T, Shibasaki H. Low-frequency repetitive transcranial magnetic stimulation for seizure suppression in patients with extratemporal lobe epilepsy - A pilot study. Seizure. 2005;**14**(6):387-392

[73] Lefaucheur JP et al. Evidence-based guidelines on the therapeutic use of repetitive transcranial magnetic stimulation (rTMS): An update (2014-2018). Clinical Neurophysiology. 2020;**131**(2):474-528

[74] George MS, Lisanby SH, Sackeim HA. Transcranial magnetic stimulation: Applications in neuropsychiatry. Archives of general psychiatry. 1999 Apr 1;**56**(4):300-311

[75] Tsuboyama M, Kaye HL, Rotenberg A. Review of transcranial magnetic stimulation in epilepsy. Clinical Therapeutics. 2020;**42**(7):1155-1168

[76] Tsuboyama M, Lee Kaye H, Rotenberg A. Biomarkers obtained by transcranial magnetic stimulation of the motor cortex in epilepsy. Frontiers in Integrated Neuroscience. 2019;**13**(October):1-10

[77] Bauer PR, De Goede AA, Ter Braack EM, Van Putten MJAM, Gill RD, Sander JW. Transcranial magnetic stimulation as a biomarker for epilepsy. Brain. 2017;**140**(3):10-12

[78] Bubrick EJ, McDannold NJ, White PJ. Low intensity focused ultrasound for Epilepsy-A new approach to neuromodulation. Epilepsy Currents. 2022 Mar 29:15357597221086111

[79] Lee CC et al. Pilot study of focused ultrasound for drug-resistant epilepsy. Epilepsia. 2022;**63**(1):162-175

[80] Tyler WJ, Tufail Y, Finsterwald M, Tauchmann ML, Olson EJ, Majestic C. Remote excitation of neuronal circuits using low-intensity, low-frequency ultrasound. PLoS One. 2008;**3**(10)

[81] Zou J, Meng L, Lin Z, Qiao Y, Tie C, Wang Y, et al. Ultrasound neuromodulation inhibits seizures in acute epileptic monkeys. Iscience. 2020 May 22;**23**(5):101066

[82] Monteith S, Snell J, Eames M, Kassell NF, Kelly E, Gwinn R. Transcranial magnetic resonance-guided focused ultrasound for temporal lobe epilepsy: A laboratory feasibility study. Journal of Neurosurgery. 2016;**125**(6):1557-1564

[83] Abe K et al. Magnetic resonance-guided focused ultrasound for mesial temporal lobe epilepsy: A case report. BMC Neurology. 2020;**20**(1):1-7

[84] Stern JM et al. Safety of focused ultrasound neuromodulation in humans with temporal lobe epilepsy. Brain Stimulation. 2021;**14**(4):1022-1031

[85] Baek H, Lockwood D, Mason EJ, Obusez E, Poturalski M, Rammo R, et al. Clinical intervention using focused ultrasound (FUS) stimulation of the brain in diverse neurological disorders. Frontiers in Neurology. 2022 May 9;**13**:880814. DOI: 10.3389/fneur.2022.880814. PMID: 35614924; PMCID: PMC9124976

Chapter 6

Pediatric Epilepsy in West Africa: Prevalence, Causes, and Management

Rhoda Olowe Taiwo and Tawfeeq Shekh-Ahmad

Abstract

Epilepsy is a neurological disorder affecting over 50 million people worldwide. Global epilepsy prevalence has been reported to be the greatest in Africa, prevalent among children living in resource-poor areas compared with all other continents. In West Africa, a meta-analysis of epilepsy prevalence was quoted to be 13–15 per 1000 persons. As a result of the lack of specialists and electroencephalographic facilities, the type of seizures that are more likely reported in rural areas is generalized tonic-clonic seizures. A high prevalence of epilepsy in low- and middle-income countries has been identified with CNS infections due to viral, bacterial, and parasitic infections. Parasitic infections including malaria, onchocerciasis, cysticercosis, and toxocariasis are believed to account for up to 27% of pediatric epilepsy cases reported in Sub-Saharan Africa, of which onchocerciasis has been more documented as a parasitic cause of epilepsy in most of west Africa. The management of epilepsy in West Africa centers around the administration of anti-seizure medications when available, and an onchocerciasis control program that has reduced onchocerciasis-associated epilepsy in these countries. However, several management options put in place still seem insufficient to curb the disease prevalence, hence improved strategy for effective control of parasite-induced epilepsy in West Africa.

Keywords: epilepsy, pediatric, West Africa, prevalence, parasites, general tonic-clonic seizures

1. Introduction

Epilepsy is a neurological condition affecting over 50 million people worldwide. It is characterized by recurrent seizures, following abnormal or excessive neuronal activities in the brain [1], representing a considerable healthcare burden with greater drug resistance and worse clinical outcomes than many other neurological diseases [2, 3]. It remains a global burden that knows no geographic, regional, or racial boundaries, occurring in men and women and affecting people of all ages, though more frequently affecting young people in the first two decades of life [4]. The prevalence of epilepsy has been reported to be greatest in Africa accounting for 37% of the global epilepsy burden compared to all other continents, as it has been acknowledged that more than 80% of people with epilepsy live in developing countries [5]. Typically, in Africa, the majority of people with epilepsy suffer from the disease from childhood, usually during their first few years of life. Mounting evidence from across five sites in Africa, suggested that over 60% of people with active convulsive seizures experience their first recorded seizure before age 13 [4, 6]. As a result of a lack of specialists, neurologists and electroencephalographic facilities, the type of seizures that are more likely reported in rural areas of Africa is the generalized tonic-clonic seizures (averaging 67% of individuals), because of the conspicuous presentation manifested, while partial seizures (averaging 8%) are most likely underestimated giving that their early stages recognitions are clinically difficult [7]. Although effective antiepileptic drugs are available, however, a substantial treatment gap is more evident in developing countries, mainly as a result of limited human and financial resources for diagnosis and treatment, cumulating in inadequate treatment in many cases [5]. Similarly, about 60% of patients with epilepsy receive no antiepileptic treatment, also for economic and social reasons [8]. Unfortunately, it is common that people with epilepsy left untreated to be faced with devastating social consequences, including stigma, discrimination, premature mortality, and reduced life chances for adults in terms of employment and marriage [9]. Here, we report the possible causes, prevalence, and management of pediatric epilepsy in West Africa.

2. Causes

Numerous causes have been attributed to the development of epilepsy in Africa and therefore it has been perceived that the origin of epilepsy is considered multidimensional in nature [10]. In a couple of decades ago, early knowledge of the etiology of epilepsy in most African countries has long been attributed to beliefs and spiritual reasons including spiritual attack, witchcraft, and other supernatural causes [11]. Moreover, as epidemiological studies in Africa progressed, knowledge of epilepsy prevalence begins to override beliefs, norms, and notions about epilepsy disease, highlighting other causes that might be contributory to the cause of pediatric epilepsy including obstetric injuries, frequent febrile convulsions, head trauma, and meningitis [10]. However, these aforementioned causes are only identified in less than 1% of epilepsy cases. In high-income countries, the main causes of epilepsy have been attributed to traumatic head/brain injuries and strokes [12, 13]. Whereas the high prevalence of epilepsy in low- and middle-income countries has been majorly identified with central nervous system (CNS) infections due to viral, bacterial, and parasitic infections [14].

Moreover, in recent times, the association between several parasitic diseases and epilepsy has gained new insights. Parasitic infection which remains the commonest cause of central nervous system infection and cause of symptomatic epilepsy; is believed to account for up to 27% of pediatric epilepsy cases reported in sub-saharan Africa, inclusive of West Africa [15]. Thus, updating an understanding of the etiology and epidemiology of epilepsy in West Africa. In addition, Africa has the highest burden of parasitic infections, which are associated with the development of epilepsy [16]. Among these parasitic infections are malaria, onchocerciasis, cysticercosis, and toxocariasis, infections with these organisms have been associated with epilepsy and are ubiquitous in Africa [15, 17–19].

2.1 Malaria

Malaria is one of the tropical parasitic diseases commonly thought to have a role in the development of epilepsy [20]. Majorly, most acute seizures are suggested to be caused by the malaria parasite *Plasmodium falciparum* (*P. falciparum*), usually in malaria-endemic areas, and these parasites are common in sub-Saharan Africa among people with epilepsy.

2.1.1 The cell cycle of malaria

Malaria parasites are mainly transmitted by a female anopheles mosquito. The parasite life cycle consists of a vector and human exoerythrocytic (hepatic) and erythrocytic stages [21]. The female mosquito (vector) bites the host during a blood meal, injecting mature sporozoites from its salivary glands into the host's bloodstream. These rapidly enter the liver hepatocytes and begin tissue schizogony-like asexual reproduction and proliferation (exoerythrocytic stage). Thereafter, thousands of merozoites are released into the bloodstream as the tissue schizonts burst the infected hepatocytes. The merozoites invade the erythrocytes, go through several asexual multiplication cycles (the erythrocytic stage), and then create new infectious merozoites that burst the erythrocytes to start a new infective cycle. In the long run, the parasite invades the CNS and causes some disruption of the BBB function, leading to cerebral malaria [22, 23].

Cerebral malaria is the most serious neurological complication of Plasmodium falciparum infection. In most infected children, after 1–3 days of fever, coma develops rapidly and seizures set in [24]. A defining feature of cerebral malaria is the Intravascular sequestration of circulating parasitized erythrocytes in the cerebral microcirculation.

Sequestration is a result of cytoadherence of infected erythrocytes to the vascular endothelial cells through parasite-derived proteins on the surfaces of the infected erythrocytes for example, the Plasmodium falciparum erythrocyte membrane protein-1 (PfEMP1) [25]. These are considered important pathophysiological mechanisms underlining cerebral malaria.

Furthermore, malaria can also cause different forms of seizures in the CNS, and it has already been identified as the most common cause of febrile seizures [26]. Agbéré et al., [27], reported that most febrile seizure cases occur in 55% of patients with malaria fever in Togo. Although the role of malaria in long-term epilepsy is still unclear, Preliminary studies have attributed a high risk of epilepsy to cerebral malaria, as seizures are one of the hallmarks of the clinical presentation of cerebral malaria [28]. An earlier study reporting an association between falciparum malaria and epilepsy found a 9% (4·4, 1·4–13·7) epilepsy occurrence in children exposed to cerebral malaria and 12% (6·1, 2·0–18·3) in those exposed to malaria and complex seizures [19]. However, whether they are febrile or acute symptomatic seizures, remains unclear [25, 29, 30].

2.2 Onchocerciasis

Human Onchocerciasis also referred to as "river blindness" caused by the filarial nematode; *Onchocerca volvulus* (*O. volvulus*), is a chronic parasitic infection transmitted by bites of blackflies [31]. Onchocerciasis is known as a cause of skin and eye disease infecting a great number of people and has also been implicated in seizure disorders mainly in rural Africa. It is estimated that of the 120 million infected, 99% of them live in Africa [32].

2.2.1 The cell cycle of onchocerciasis

Several mechanisms have been proposed for the pathogenesis of onchocerciasis-related epilepsy. However, one of the most identified mechanisms is the *O. volvulus*-induced immune response via an inflammatory process or autoantibodies against neuron surface proteins such as the voltage-gated potassium channel complex (VGKC), the N-methyl-D-aspartate (NMDA), a-amino-3-hydroxy-5-methyl-4-isoxazole propionic acid (AMPA), gamma-aminobutyric acid (GABA)A, GABAB, and glycine receptors which are recognized causes of severe epileptic disorders [33].

Similarly, *Wolbachia* which are intracytoplasmic symbiotic bacteria found in filarial worms' endosymbiont of *O. volvulus* has also been proposed as a possible cause of onchocerciasis-related epilepsy. *O. volvulus* endemic areas, is a neuroinflammatory disorder caused by antibodies to either *O. volvulus* or its co-symbiotic bacteria, Wolbachia, cross-reacting with host neuron surface proteins, although evidence for neuroinflammation has not been established [34].

Consistent reports from epidemiological studies suggest that *O. volvulus* infection is a trigger and risk factor for epilepsy in Onchocerca endemic areas [35]. In Africa, onchocerciasis-associated epilepsy (OAE) was first documented in a population-based epidemiological study in the Mbam valley in Cameroon between 1991 and 1992, where high epilepsy prevalence was associated with communities near Mbam River, a breeding site for black flies [36].

In addition, several studies have reported an association between the prevalence of onchocerciasis and epilepsy in different areas of east, west, and central Africa [36–38]. In West Africa, epidemiological studies have identified a high prevalence of epilepsy to a high onchocerciasis endemicity, where most infected patients experience generalized tonic-clonic seizures and the risk for children developing epilepsy has been determined by the *O. volvulus* microfilariae load [35, 39]. Although a paucity of information has been reported on *O. volvulus* penetration to the CNS, nonetheless, the presence of microfilariae from various filarial species in the human CNS has been reported. Studies suggest that since antifilariae drugs can provoke the passage of Loa Loa microfilariae (responsible for spontaneous encephalitis) into the cerebrospinal fluid (CSF) [40], therefore it does seem that *O. volvulus* would be able to penetrate the CNS since microfilariae belonging to this species have been found in the CSF of Onchocerciasis patients with or without filaricidal drugs [41, 42]. Furthermore, another explanation that *O. volvulus* could directly or indirectly cause epilepsy could be the occurrence of antibody-mediated autoinflammatory response against *O. volvulus*, cross-reacting with neuronal proteins [43] (**Figure 1**), as antibodies to voltage-gated potassium channels in neurons have recently been observed [44]. However, irrespective of this attribute, the pathophysiological mechanisms involved in onchocerciasis associated with epilepsy for seizure induction still need to be further elucidated.

2.3 Neurocysticercosis

Neurocysticercosis (Cysticercosis), remains the commonest helminthic infection of the CNS, representing an important cause of secondary epilepsy globally

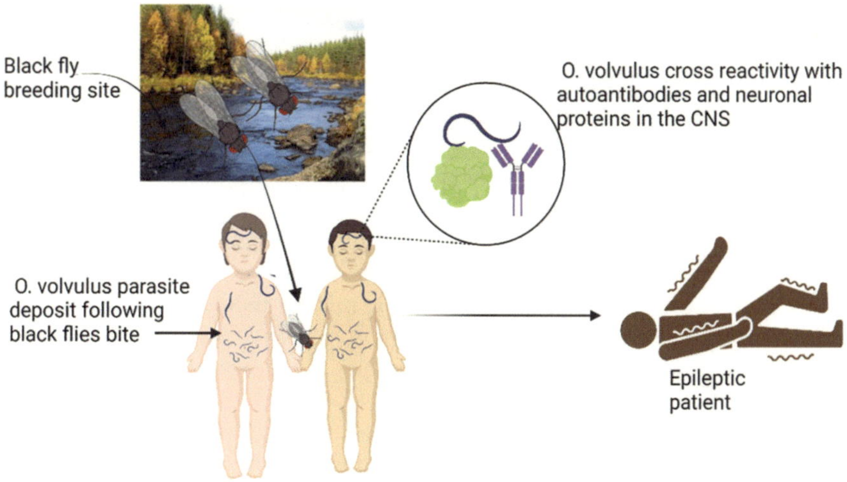

Figure 1.
The postulated scenario of infection or events of onchocerciasis associated epilepsy (AOE).

[45, 46]. It is a cause of epilepsy in some parts of the world, and the introduction of computed tomography (CT) in the 1970s and early 1980s has allowed for its detection [47]. Cysticercosis is regarded as a Zoonotic disease, commonly caused by the larval stage (cysticercus) of the porcine tapeworm *Taenia Solium* (*T. solium*) and is said to be mainly found in the CNS including the Brain and spines. Reports of the parasite development in the brain, suggest an appearance of immature cysticerci in the brain within some weeks after ingestion of *T. Solium* eggs [48, 49].

2.3.1 The cell cycle of neurocysticercosis

In a typical life cycle of *T.* solium, following ingestion of the parasite, the adult worm is found in the small intestine of humans (the sole definite host of the parasite). The worms produce per day tens of thousands of oncospheres (eggs), They are then eliminated via feces, contaminating the food chain and water systems. Pigs (intermediate hosts of parasites) consume these oncospheres, where they are activated by bile salts and digestive enzymes in the small intestine. They subsequently go into the blood supply through the gut wall at blood vessel terminations in a variety of tissues (such as muscle, subcutaneous tissue, or nerve tissue) [50]. When a human consumes improperly cooked pork that contains a cysticercus, the scolex evaginates in the small intestine and clings to the intestinal wall where it develops into an adult worm.

However, when a person accidentally becomes an intermediate host and consumes oncospheres via tainted food or water, the oncospheres are thereafter activated in the human digestive tract just as they are in the pig, allowing them to pass into the bloodstream. They embed themselves in a variety of tissues, particularly the central nervous system. Taenia *solium* cysticerci invade and infect the brain parenchyma, of which seizures are the most common manifestation of parenchyma disease [51]. When cysticerci are present in the nervous system this is referred to as neurocysticercosis (NCC).

Although this parasite is mainly reported to cause 20–50% of all late-onset cases of epilepsy globally. Moreover, in a certain part of the world, it is assumed to be a common cause of juvenile epilepsy, majorly in the southern part of Africa [52, 53].

Nonetheless, this infection has been under-recognized in many developing countries, certainly true for Africa and more specifically West Africa, where this infection has been only reported in a few countries [47]. For instance, it is rarely reported in Nigeria unlike her neighboring countries, Cameroun, Benin, and Togo, where cysticercosis-associated epilepsy showed a significant proportion of epilepsy cases [54]. In an epidemiological study in Togo, cysticercosis prevalence was 135% among people with epilepsy (PWE) compared to 38% of the general population [55]. However, the high prevalence of neurocysticercosis is streamed lined to the rural area where a high consumption of pork infected with *T. Solium* predisposes people to epilepsy, resulting in one of the main causes of acquired epilepsy in middle-income countries around sub-Saharan Africa, inclusive of West Africa [45].

2.4 Toxocariasis

Human toxocariasis is another most prevalent helminthiasis also regarded as a parasitic zoonosis caused by the larval stages of dogs roundworm; *Toxocara canis* (*T. canis*), and by roundworm of cats; *Toxocara cati* (*T. cati*) [56]. Infections are mainly established through direct contact with the animals or via ingestion of contaminated food. Upon ingestion, eggs metamorphose into juvenile larvae capable of crossing the small intestine into the systemic circulation and then migrate to organs particularly muscles, and at times to the CNS where they invoke multisystemic inflammatory reactions [57].

2.4.1 The cell cycle of toxocariasis

The gastrointestinal ascarid nematodes Toxocara spp., including *T.* canis and *T. cati*, are present in canids (definitive hosts), such as dogs, felids (domestic cats), as well as foxes, and jackals. They can also infect people (considered paratenic hosts) through direct contact with diseased cats and dogs as well as contaminated food, soil, and water, of which humans tend to unintentionally consume eggs containing infectious third-stage larvae [58, 59].

Eggs that have been consumed grow and hatch into larvae in the small intestine, pierce the intestinal wall, and move through the circulatory system to various tissues. This causes an immune and inflammatory tissue reaction, which can cause symptoms like fever, headaches, coughing, and abdominal or limb pains [59].

Neurotoxocariasis, also known as cerebral toxocariasis, resulting from toxocara larvae invades the brain. In the brain, the larvae can also induce epileptic convulsions, cerebral vasculitis, and eosinophilic meningitis. Similarly, reports from experimental animal models showed that the presence of Toxocara larvae in the brain leads to neuronal damage via an increase in BBB permeability, expression of proinflammatory cytokines, iNOS, and astrogliosis [60, 61]. In addition, there have also been reports of changes in the profiles of neurotransmitters such as GABA, glutamate, serotonin, dopamine, and noradrenaline [62].

In nutshell, Toxocara larvae can invade the CNS by crossing the blood-brain barrier resulting in neurotoxocariasis [63]. Seroprevalence of the parasite tends to reach up to 80–90% in tropical regions, including West Africa while seroprevalence in western countries ranges from 35 to 42% and 2 to 5% in rural and urban areas, respectively [60]. Early epidemiological studies have provided evidence of a positive association between Toxocara seropositivity and seizure in children. Arpino et al., [64], evaluated the relationship between toxocariasis infection and epilepsy in children and reported that a significant ($p < 0.05$) association existed between seropositivity for anti-Toxocara canis and seizures and this correlation was closest in children below age five. Furthermore, an investigation on the possible association between epilepsy and toxocariasis in the kiremba population of Burundi revealed that out of the studied 191 PWE, antibodies of anti-*T. canis* were found in 114 PWE (59.7%) and multivariate analysis showed a significant association between positivity for *T.* canis and epilepsy [65]. Although, some studies have proven an association. However, reports from two other studies revealed a non-significant association between epilepsy and seropositivity (antitoxocaral antibodies) [66, 67], adding up a piece of conflicting evidence that is difficult to interpret. To gain more insights into the association of this parasite with epilepsy, further studies are necessary to clarify its potential role and activity in epilepsy.

3. Prevalence

Reports have shown that the prevalence of epilepsy is higher in less developed than in more developed countries, with prevalence estimated from door-to-door studies almost double that in Asia, Europe, and North America [45]. More precisely, in West Africa, a meta-analysis of epilepsy prevalence was quoted to be between 13.14 and 15 per 1000 persons. However, this incidence has been more prevalent among children living in resource-poor (rural) areas than in urban areas [31]. The region-specific prevalence of epilepsy has yielded a treatment gap, resulting from inadequate access to physicians trained to manage epilepsy, a lack of access to ASM, poor knowledge about epilepsy among the communities, as well as the stigma of epilepsy arising from misconceptions about; epilepsy having a supernatural origin and attributed to possession by ancestral spirits [68]. In addition, the stigma of epilepsy can be profound because it is widely thought to be contagious and associated with witchcraft [69]. This stigma surrounding the disease creates psychosocial impacts on the children, marginalizing their ability to participate in community/societal activities leading to a significant effect on their quality of life [70].

Although a paucity of information has been gathered on epilepsy prevalence in West Africa, nonetheless several studies have reported a higher occurrence of epilepsy in onchocerciasis-endemic sites across countries in West Africa. In Nigeria, epilepsy prevalence based on defined communities varies between 15 and 37 per 1000 [31, 71]. An early epidemiological survey investigating the possible relationship of epilepsy with onchocerciasis in towns and villages in Nigeria observed a 37% epilepsy prevalence in Aiyete; a rural onchocerciasis-endemic village [72] while in Igbo-Ora; a town inhabited by the same ethnic group as Aiyete, situated 20 km away recorded 5.3% epilepsy prevalence, in the age group between 10 and 19 years [72, 73]. The lower prevalence recorded in Igbo-Ora compared to Aiyete may be due to the availability of comprehensive health facilities, effective primary health care with greater emphasis on antenatal care, improved prevention of childhood infectious diseases, and a working health education system [72]. Moreover, Aiyete is said to be located closer to the Ofiki River, a known breeding site for blackflies, causing this village to pose a higher endemicity than Igbo-Ora [74]. Furthermore, in a study carried out on 13 villages in the Imo River basin; a southeastern part of Nigeria that is mesoendemic for onchocerciasis, reports revealed a 12% epilepsy prevalence in these villages with a higher prevalence of onchocerciasis ranging between 8.3 and 36% and higher microfilariae density [39].

Furthermore, epilepsy prevalence reports in Benin; a country bordering Nigeria to the west revealed that 9/13 (69.2%) PWE in the Agbome area were associated with O. volvulus microfilariae which were detected in skin snips while 8 PWE (61.5%) presented with onchocerciasis nodules. In addition, the majority of these patients (76.9%) manifested generalized tonic-clonic seizures [75].

In Ghana, albeit a community-based survey of kintampo village, revealed a lower epilepsy prevalence of as low as 1.92%, the epilepsy cases were attributed to exposure to O. volvulus and were identified as an independent risk factor for epilepsy in children below 18 years [76].

Furthermore, in Mali, epidemiological studies conducted on the endemicity of onchocerciasis about epilepsy prevalence in 18 villages showed an epilepsy prevalence of 16.1 per 1000 in zones of high endemicity of onchocerciasis (23.0%) compared to a prevalence of 10.8 per 1000 in zones of low endemicity (9.3%). Although a non-significant difference was reported between these two zones, however, higher morbidity rates were reported in zones of high endemicity of onchocerciasis [77].

In Cameroon, an outcome of a clinical epilepsy prevalence survey of 156 PWE in selected 5 onchocerciasis-endemic villages, revealed that onchocerciasis-associated epilepsy (OAE) showed a high prevalence in epilepsy patients where 93.2% of PWE met the criteria for OAE, presenting with the most frequent seizure types being generalized tonic-clonic episodes, absences, and nodding seizures. More so, the majority of epilepsies started between the ages of 3 and 18 years [78].

In epilepsy prevalence studies in Liberia, two studies documented a high epilepsy prevalence of 27.73–49.01% in Grad Bassa, which was agreed that the prevalence was in an onchocerciasis endemic area [79, 80].

In Ivory Coast, an epidemiological survey carried out in a village less than 10 km from M'Brou, where a high burden of epilepsy had previously been reported for decades with a microfilariae prevalence of 76%, revealed an epilepsy prevalence of 41% (38 of 920) and 73.7% fulfilled the OAE criteria [81].

In Burkina Faso, a prevalence study of epilepsy in three villages has specifically identified epilepsy prevalence with a positive reaction to cysticercosis Ag-ELISA serology with an association with past pork consumption. The findings reported that 39 of 70 that screened positive for cysticercosis were confirmed to have epilepsy, suggesting the presence of neurocysticercosis as the cause of epilepsy. Collectively, a total of 70 (7.9%) of 888 persons interviewed for epilepsy or seizure screened positive and 29 (74.4%) were reported to have experienced generalized seizures [82].

Epilepsy prevalence in almost all study sites in Togo was reported to be below 20%, however, these epilepsies were said to be associated with cysticercosis, where its prevalence was 135% among PWE compared to 38% of the whole population [83]. In addition, an epilepsy management study in the Batamariba district of Togo revealed an epilepsy prevalence estimation of 15.7% of 98 patients, where the etiologies of 14/98 PWE (14.3%) were confirmed to be associated with neurocysticercosis (subcutaneous cysticercus cyst) [55]. However, in rural Gambia, a lower active epilepsy prevalence of 4.3/1000 was reported which is non-endemic for neither Neurocysticercosis nor onchocerciasis. In patients whose etiology could be suggested, etiology was only attributed to febrile illness in childhood and antenatal or perinatal brain insult [84].

Similarly, in Senegal, in the early 60s, a lower epilepsy prevalence of 1.92% was reported in an area non-endemic for onchocerciasis located in the Moyenne Vallée of Senegal. However, a more recent study from Pikine Health District of Senegal reported an epilepsy prevalence of 14.22% also in a non-endemic area [85].

Country	Towns/Villages	Causative parasite	Prevalence	Reference
Nigeria	Ayete	Onchocerciasis	37%	[72]
Nigeria	Igbo ora	Onchocerciasis	5.9%	[72, 73]
Nigeria	Imo	Onchocerciasis	12%	[39]
Benin	Agbome	Onchocerciasis	69.2%	[75]
Ghana	Kintampo	Onchocerciasis	1.92%	[76]
Mali	18 pooled villages	Onchocerciasis	16.1%	[77]
Liberia	Grad Bassa	Onchocerciasis	27.73–49.01%	[79, 80]
Cameroon	5 pooled villages	Onchocerciasis	93.2%	[78]
Ivory Coast	M'brou	Onchocerciasis	41%	[81]
Burkinafaso	3 pooled villages	Neurocysticercosis	7.9%	[82]
Togo	Batamariba	Neurocycticercosis	15.7%	[55]
The Gambia	Farafenni	Febrile Seizure	<1%	[84]
Senegal	Moyenne valle	NA	1.92%	[85]
Senegal	Pikine	NA	14.2%	[85]

NA-Not applicable.

Table 1.
Summary of identified prevalence and cause of epilepsy in west African countries.

The majority of these findings strongly incriminate onchocerciasis as an important yet neglected contributor to the epilepsy burden in West Africa (**Table 1**).

4. Management

Management of Epilepsy in West Africa centers around the administration of ASM to control seizures as epilepsy surgery is rarely available in most parts of Africa [86]. However, in rural areas, a wide treatment gap is usually reported, and a systemic review has identified several reasons for this treatment gap including scarcity of knowledgeable staff, lack of investigative resources to ensure a diagnosis, cost of treatment, far-flung distance to health care facilities, cultural beliefs and inadequate availability of anti-seizure medications [87]. The presence of treatment gaps in West Africa has accounted for a high mortality rate related to poorly controlled epilepsy, with a greater proportion of children dying from status epilepticus compared to other continents [88]. In addition, in a systematic review, the World Health Organization (WHO) reported a greater treatment gap of 95% in some African countries including Ethiopia, Nigeria, Togo, Uganda, Tanzania, Gambia, and Zambia [89]. In most developing countries, available medications in the treatment and management of partial seizures include but are not limited to Carbamazepine, Phenobarbital, and Phenytoin, while drugs of choice for patients with tonic-clonic seizures are Valproic acid and Phenobarbital [90, 91]. However, Phenobarbital is the single most commonly prescribed anti-seizure medication for reasons due to availability, economic considerations, and its effectiveness in reducing the frequency of partial and generalized tonic-clonic seizures [92]. Moreover, the WHO has recommended Phenobarbital as the first-line therapy for convulsive epilepsy in Africa since it's the most readily available and cost-effective ASM for seizure management [93]. Furthermore, another management practice particularly influenced by the introduction of the vector control program, that has been deployed in West Africa is the OCP (1974–2002), executed through a largescale onchocerciasis elimination control measure, followed by annual microfilaricidal treatment with Ivermectin distribution [94]. These control measures have significantly reduced OAE and drastically decrease the incidence of epilepsy in 11 countries in West Africa [95, 96]. However, despite the documented success, several challenges remain unmet, including banishing the stigma associated with epilepsy and dealing with cultural and social beliefs culminating in poor help-seeking behaviors among family and community of epilepsy patients. Ensuring easy access to anti-seizure medications at a cheaper or subsidized cost; Improving sensitization on relying on the primary health care system for treatments in rural areas.

5. Discussion

In most developing countries like West Africa, epilepsy disease remains prevalent in the younger population of resource-deprived communities. The majority of epidemiological studies indicate that the age of epilepsy onset is younger in underdeveloped countries than in areas with greater access to resources [97]. The survey methodology commonly employed in population studies of epilepsy is the door-to-door epidemiological survey, where a questionnaire is provided to screen members of a household with epilepsy [98].

However, this survey method poses a likely problem of underestimation as the screening tends to identify majorly individuals with generalized tonic-clonic seizure, and under-recognition is given to individuals with partial complex, dyscognitive, or myoclonic seizures, thereby underestimating the prevalence of the disease [99]. Additionally, people who have children with epilepsy tend not to declare the condition in a bid to avoid epilepsy-associated stigmas. The stigma attached to epilepsy may make people reluctant to acknowledge that someone in their home has the illness, thus resulting in the unavailability of epidemiological data [45].

Although, about three decades ago, epilepsy patients are rarely stigmatized because the condition is believed to be of demonic origin, attributed as being possessed and it is only combated with sorcery and traditional medicines with no seeming solutions [72, 73]. Just in recent times, following community sensitization about the disease condition and communities were enlightened on the disease being of medical origin, identified as epilepsy, bringing about the stigmatization of the disease. It is commonly established that epilepsy stigma has an impact on many aspects of its victim's life, such as social isolation, low self-esteem, worse psychological function, and increased future uncertainty [100]. Nonetheless, a well establishes effective epilepsy enlightenment campaign, as well as epilepsy education, could help patients and their families have comprehensive information on epilepsy disorder, avoid misconceptions and overcome the challenge of stigma in the resource-poor areas where epilepsy prevalence is pronounced [101].

Moreover, it is known that 80% of people with epilepsy reside in resource-poor, developing countries, however, a huge treatment gap exists, where epilepsy care in these regions remains limited and a majority of epilepsy patients go untreated [8]. Treatment gaps resulting from weak healthcare structures, inadequate financial resources, unreliable supply and quality of pharmaceuticals, the high rate of inappropriate self-medication, unavailability of ASM, inadequate ASM storage conditions are likely to lead to ineffective and possibly dangerous ASMs [102], and even when good-quality ASMs are initially imported. Highlighting the difficulties with antiepileptics and, indeed, all drug use in developing countries [103].

To overcome these challenges, sustainable epilepsy care services that can deliver first-line antiepileptic drugs through established primary healthcare facilities, are needed to reduce these treatment gaps. Furthermore, Neurologists with knowledge of the culture and local experiences, who are willing to serve as advocates, educators, and policy advisors, can help make a difference. Nonetheless, a more sophisticated approach to overcoming the hurdles of epilepsy treatment in resource-poor nations is the availability of expertise for reliable EEG video interpretation of different seizure types for effective treatment and the establishment of a sustainable epilepsy monitor program.

6. Conclusions

Epilepsy in West Africa remains an undebatable challenge majorly in children in their first few years of life. Knowing fully that prevalence studies are a prerequisite for successful intervention. The primary purpose of this report was to assess the prevalence, causes, and management of pediatric epilepsy in West African countries at a community level and to bring to the limelight the available knowledge with previously existing data on this subject that dates way back to over 3 decades ago. We have recalled a parasitic cause of epilepsy that has been the main concern in tropical countries like West Africa. Parasitic infections including malaria, onchocerciasis, cysticercosis, and toxocariasis remain a common cause of CNS infection and cause of symptomatic epilepsy; where onchocerciasis is believed to account for up to 27% of pediatric epilepsy cases. These findings strongly incriminate onchocerciasis as an important yet neglected contributor to epilepsy in West Africa. Parasite-induced epilepsy remains a burden in many parts of West Africa, where generalized tonic-clonic and partial seizures were the predominant seizure types that have been reported. So far, the main achievements in dealing with epilepsy in West Africa involve the administration of available ASM such as Carbamazepine, Phenobarbital, Valproic acid, and Phenytoin, albeit a wide treatment gap is usually reported. Currently, resource-poor communities in low-income nations are unable to fund desirable but expensive initiatives like specialized epilepsy centers, which would appear to be the best method to assist epileptic patients in poor nations. Nonetheless, subsidized antiseizure medications could be provided to community health care centers so as to be at the disposal of the patients. More so, a national organization that is associated with international organizations for epilepsy could solicit and receive support and encouragement from international bodies like the International Bureau of Epilepsy. In addition, the introduction of the onchocerciasis control program has been deployed in West Africa as a parasitic control measure for onchocerciasis-induced seizures.

However, pediatric epilepsy in West Africa has long been underestimated as a paucity of information has only been gathered so far on its prevalence, causes, and management. It could be a result of the lower number of epidemiological studies carried out, arising from the stigma attached to epilepsy, as some people still hide the diagnosis; hence contributing to the underestimated prevalence of the disease. To overcome this challenge, education relevant to epilepsy health education such as patient-centered care allows individuals with epilepsy and their families to access usable information including Knowledge of epilepsy in general, an explanation of what happens during a seizure, and the importance of getting medical help, the significance of trigger factors that may induce a seizure, a guide to ASMs; how they work, their side effects and the importance of compliance, orientations on improved quality of life, managing lifestyle and wellness should be encouraged at all levels to debunk wrong notions and myths about epilepsy as well to control the stigmatization of affected people. Furthermore, more epidemiological studies for improved interventions are required.

Acknowledgements

The authors are thankful to The Neubauer Family Foundation for their generous support of our research.

We also acknowledge the David R. Bloom Center for Pharmacy for financial support. The research also received support from The Israel Science Foundation (grant no. 1976/20 to TSA).

Conflict of interest

The authors declare no conflict of interest.

Acronyms and abbreviations

ASM	Anti-seizure medication
CNS	Central nervous system
CSF	Cerebrospinal fluid
CT	Computed tomography
OAE	Onchocerciasis associated epilepsy
OCP	Onchocerciasis control program
BBB	Blood-Brain-Barrier
PWE	People with epilepsy
P. falciparum	Plasmodium falciparum
T. canis	Toxocara *Canis*
T. cati	Toxocara *cati*
O. volvulus	Onchocerca *volvulus*
T. solium	Taenia solium
WHO	World Health Organization

Author details

Rhoda Olowe Taiwo and Tawfeeq Shekh-Ahmad*
The Institute for Drug Research, The School of Pharmacy, Faculty of Medicine, The Hebrew University of Jerusalem, Jerusalem, Israel

*Address all correspondence to: tawfeeq.shekh-ahmad@mail.huji.ac.il

References

[1] Huang LG, Zou J, Lu QC. Silencing rno-miR-155-5p in rat temporal lobe epilepsy model reduces pathophysiological features and cell apoptosis by activating Sestrin-3. Brain Research. 2018;**1689**:109-122

[2] Sun H, Ma L, Zhang Y, Pan X, Wang C, Zhang J, et al. A purinergic P2 receptor family-mediated increase in Thrombospondin-1 bolsters synaptic density and epileptic seizure activity in the amygdala-kindling rat model. Frontiers in Cellular Neuroscience. 2018;**12**:302

[3] Zhang Y, Zhang M, Zhu W, Yu J, Wang Q, Zhang J, et al. Succinate accumulation induces mitochondrial reactive oxygen species generation and promotes status epilepticus in the kainic acid rat model. Redox Biology. 2020;**28**:101365

[4] Sander JW. The epidemiology of epilepsy revisited. Current Opinion in Neurology. 2003;**16**(2):165-170

[5] Meinardi H, Scott RA, Reis R, Sander JWAS, World ICD. The treatment gap in epilepsy: The current situation and ways forward. Epilepsia. 2001;**42**(1):136-149

[6] Duncan JS, Sander JW, Sisodiya SM, Walker MC. Adult epilepsy. Lancet. 2006;**367**(9516):1087-1100

[7] Kaiser C, Benninger C, Asaba G, Mugisa C, Kabagambe G, Kipp W, et al. Clinical and electro-clinical classification of epileptic seizure in West Uganda. Bulletin de la Societe de Pathologie Exotique. 2000;**93**(4):255-259

[8] Ngugi AK, Bottomley C, Kleinschmidt I, Sander JW, Newton CR. Estimation of the burden of active and life-time epilepsy: A meta-analytic approach. Epilepsia. 2010;**51**(5):883-890

[9] Vos T, Flaxman AD, Naghavi M, Lozano R, Michaud C, Ezzati M, et al. Years lived with disability (YLDs) for 1160 sequelae of 289 diseases and injuries 1990-2010: A systematic analysis for the global burden of disease study 2010. Lancet. 2012;**380**(9859):2163-2196

[10] Osakwe C, Otte WM, Alo C. Epilepsy prevalence, potential causes and social beliefs in Ebonyi state and Benue state, Nigeria. Epilepsy Research. 2014;**108**(2):316-326

[11] Komolafe M, Sunmonu T, Fabusiwa F, Komolafe E, Afolabi O, Kett M, et al. Women's perspectives on epilepsy and its sociocultural impact in south western Nigeria. African Journal of Neurological Sciences. 2011;**30**(2):39-48

[12] Garcia-Martin G, Perez-Errazquin F, Chamorro-Munoz MI, Romero-Acebal M, Martin-Reyes G, Dawid-Milner MS. Prevalence and clinical characteristics of epilepsy in the south of Spain. Epilepsy Research. 2012;**102**(1-2):100-108

[13] Rai D, Kerr MP, McManus S, Jordanova V, Lewis G, Brugha TS. Epilepsy and psychiatric comorbidity: A nationally representative population-based study. Epilepsia. 2012;**53**(6):1095-1103

[14] Forsgren L. Estimations of the prevalence of epilepsy in sub-Saharan Africa. Lancet Neurology. 2008;7(1):21-22

[15] Ngugi AK, Bottomley C, Kleinschmidt I, Wagner RG, Kakooza-Mwesige A, Ae-Ngibise K, et al.

Prevalence of active convulsive epilepsy in sub-Saharan Africa and associated risk factors: Cross-sectional and case-control studies. Lancet Neurology. 2013;**12**(3):253-263

[16] Birbeck G, Chomba E, Atadzhanov M, Mbewe E, Haworth A. The social and economic impact of epilepsy in Zambia: A cross-sectional study. Lancet Neurology. 2007;**6**(1):39-44

[17] Matuja WB, Kilonzo G, Mbena P, Mwango'mbola RL, Wong P, Goodfellow P, et al. Risk factors for epilepsy in a rural area in Tanzania. A community-based case-control study. Neuroepidemiology. 2001;**20**(4):242-247

[18] Birbeck GL. Epilepsy in Africa: Caution and optimism. Lancet Neurology. 2013;**12**(3):220-222

[19] Carter JA, Neville BG, White S, Ross AJ, Otieno G, Mturi N, et al. Increased prevalence of epilepsy associated with severe falciparum malaria in children. Epilepsia. 2004;**45**(8):978-981

[20] Ngoungou EB, Dulac O, Poudiougou B, Druet-Cabanac M, Dicko A, Traore AM, et al. Epilepsy as a consequence of cerebral malaria in the area in which malaria is endemic in Mali, West Africa. Epilepsia. 2006;**47**(5):873-879

[21] Sinka ME, Bangs MJ, Manguin S, Rubio-Palis Y, Chareonviriyaphap T, Coetzee M, et al. A global map of dominant malaria vectors. Parasites & Vectors. 2012;**5**:69

[22] Cowman AF, Healer J, Marapana D, Marsh K. Malaria: Biology and disease. Cell. 2016;**167**(3):610-624

[23] Venugopal K, Hentzschel F, Valkiūnas G, Marti M. Plasmodium asexual growth and sexual development in the haematopoietic niche of the host. Nature Reviews. Microbiology. 2020;**18**(3):177-189

[24] Idro R, Marsh K, John CC, Newton CRJ. Cerebral malaria: Mechanisms of brain injury and strategies for the improved neurocognitive outcome. Pediatric Research. 2010;**68**(4):267-274

[25] Idro R, Jenkins NE, Newton CR. Pathogenesis, clinical features, and neurological outcome of cerebral malaria. Lancet Neurology. 2005;**4**(12):827-840

[26] Waller D, Krishna S, Crawley J, Miller K, Nosten F, Chapman D, et al. Clinical features and outcome of severe malaria in Gambian children. Clinical Infectious Diseases. 1995;**21**(3):577-587

[27] Agbéré A, Tatagan K, Madikorai M, Eklu-Avlasu E, Balaka B, Bakondé B. Les crises convulsives de l'enfant dans le service de Pédiatrie du centre hospitalier régional de Kara (Nord-Togo). Médecine d'Afrique Noire. 1995;**42**(6):310-314

[28] Ngoungou EB, Druet-Cabanac M, Dulac O, Kombila M, Doumbo O, Preux P-M, editors. Cerebral malaria and epilepsy in a cohort of 322 Malian children. In: Abstract from the 25th International Epilepsy Congress, Lisbon, Portugal, 12-16 October, 2003. Vol. 44, Supplement 8. Epilepsia: Wiley Online Library; 2003. p. 60

[29] Winkler AS. Neurocysticercosis in sub-Saharan Africa: A review of prevalence, clinical characteristics, diagnosis, and management. Pathog Global Health. 2012;**106**(5):261-274

[30] Quattrocchi G, Nicoletti A, Marin B, Bruno E, Druet-Cabanac M, Preux PM. Toxocariasis and epilepsy:

Systematic review and meta-analysis. PLoS Neglected Tropical Diseases. 2012;**6**(8):e1775

[31] Siewe Fodjo JN, Remme JHF, Preux PM, Colebunders R. Meta-analysis of epilepsy prevalence in West Africa and its relationship with onchocerciasis endemicity and control. International Health. 2020;**12**(3):192-202

[32] Duke BOL. Human onchocerciasis - an overview of the disease. Acta Leidensia. 1990;**59**(1-2):9-24

[33] Vincent A, Bien CG, Irani SR, Waters P. Autoantibodies associated with diseases of the CNS: New developments and future challenges. The Lancet Neurology. 2011;**10**(8):759-772

[34] Galán-Puchades MT. Onchocerciasis-associated epilepsy. The Lancet Infectious Diseases. 2019;**19**(1):21-22

[35] Chesnais CB, Nana-Djeunga HC, Njamnshi AK, Lenou-Nanga CG, Boulle C, Bissek ACZK, et al. The temporal relationship between onchocerciasis and epilepsy: A population-based cohort study. Lancet Infectious Diseases. 2018;**18**(11):1278-1286

[36] Boussinesq M, Pion SDS, Demanga-Ngangue KJ. Relationship between onchocerciasis and epilepsy: A matched case-control study in the Mbam Valley, Republic of Cameroon. Transactions of the Royal Society of Tropical Medicine and Hygiene. 2002;**96**(5):537-541

[37] Pion SD, Kaiser C, Boutros-Toni F, Cournil A, Taylor MM, Meredith SE, et al. Epilepsy in onchocerciasis endemic areas: Systematic review and meta-analysis of population-based surveys. PLoS Neglected Tropical Diseases. 2009;**3**(6):e461

[38] Pion SDS, Boussinesq M. Significant association between epilepsy and presence of Onchocercal nodules: Case-control study in Cameroon. American Journal of Tropical Medicine and Hygiene. 2012;**86**(3):557

[39] Dozie IN, Onwuliri CO, Nwoke BE, Chukwuocha UM, Chikwendu CI, Okoro I, et al. Onchocerciasis and epilepsy in parts of the Imo river basin, Nigeria: A preliminary report. Public Health. 2006;**120**(5):448-450

[40] Ducorps M, Gardon-Wendel N, Ranque S, Ndong W, Boussinesq M, Gardon J, et al. Effets secondaires du traitement de la loase hypermicrofilarémique par l'ivermectine. Bulletin Society Pathology Exotic. 1995;**88**:105-112

[41] Mazzoti L. Presencia de microfilariasis de Onchocerca volvulus en al liquids cefalorraquides de enfrmos tratados con hetrazan. Revista del Instituto Salubridad Enfermedades Tropicales Mexico. 1959;**19**:1-5

[42] Duke BO, Vincelette J, Moore PJ. Microfilariae in the cerebrospinal fluid, and neurological complications, during treatment of onchocerciasis with diethylcarbamazine. Tropenmedizin und Parasitologie. 1976;**27**(2):123-132

[43] Johnson TP, Tyagi R, Lee PR, Lee MH, Johnson KR, Kowalak J, et al. Nodding syndrome may be an autoimmune reaction to the parasitic worm Onchocerca volvulus. Science Translational Medicine. 2017;**9**(377):eaaf6953

[44] Idro R, Opar B, Wamala J, Abbo C, Onzivua S, Mwaka DA, et al. Is nodding syndrome an Onchocerca volvulus-induced neuroinflammatory disorder? Uganda's story of research in understanding the disease. International

Journal of Infectious Diseases. 2016;**45**:112-117

[45] Preux PM, Druet-Cabanac M. Epidemiology and aetiology of epilepsy in sub-Saharan Africa. Lancet Neurology. 2005;**4**(1):21-31

[46] Del Brutto OH, Santibanez R, Idrovo L, Rodriguez S, Diaz-Calderon E, Navas C, et al. Epilepsy and neurocysticercosis in Atahualpa: A door-to-door survey in rural coastal Ecuador. Epilepsia. 2005;**46**(4):583-587

[47] Zoli A, Shey-Njila O, Assana E, Nguekam JP, Dorny P, Brandt J, et al. Regional status, epidemiology and impact of Taenia solium cysticercosis in Western and Central Africa. Acta Tropica. 2003;**87**(1):35-42

[48] Carpio A, Hauser WA. Prognosis for seizure recurrence in patients with newly diagnosed neurocysticercosis. Neurology. 2002;**59**(11):1730-1734

[49] Del Brutto OH. Clinical management of neurocysticercosis. Expert Review of Neurotherapeutics. 2014;**14**(4):389-396

[50] White AC. Neurocysticercosis: Updates on epidemiology, pathogenesis, diagnosis, and management. Annual Review of Medicine. 2000;**51**(1):187-206

[51] Ndimubanzi PC, Carabin H, Budke CM, Nguyen H, Qian Y J, Rainwater E, et al. A systematic review of the frequency of neurocysticercosis with a focus on people with epilepsy. PLoS Neglected Tropical Diseases. 2010;**4**(11):e870

[52] Grill J, Rakotomalala W, Andriantsimahavandy A, Boisier P, Guyon P, Roux J, et al. High prevalence of serological markers of cysticercosis among epileptic Malagasy children. Annals of Tropical Paediatrics. 1996;**16**(3):185-191

[53] Mafojane NA, Appleton CC, Krecek RC, Michael LM, Willingham AL 3rd. The current status of neurocysticercosis in eastern and southern Africa. Acta Tropica. 2003;**87**(1):25-33

[54] Balogou A, Grunitzky K, Beketi K, Bouteille B, Dumas M. Cysticercosis and epilepsy in the city of tone, north of Togo. Revue Neurologique. 2000;**156**(3):270-273

[55] Balogou AA, Grunitzky EK, Belo M, Sankaredja M, Djagba DD, Tatagan-Agbi K, et al. Management of epilepsy patients in Batamariba district, Togo. Acta Neurologica Scandinavica. 2007;**116**(4):211-216

[56] Luna J, Cicero CE, Rateau G, Quattrocchi G, Marin B, Bruno E, et al. Updated evidence of the association between toxocariasis and epilepsy: Systematic review and meta-analysis. PLoS Neglected Tropical Diseases. 2018;**12**(7):e0006665

[57] Schantz PM, Glickman LT. Toxocaral visceral larva migrans. The New England Journal of Medicine. 1978;**298**(8):436-439

[58] Ma G, Holland CV, Wang T, Hofmann A, Fan C-K, Maizels RM, et al. Human toxocariasis. The Lancet Infectious Diseases. 2018;**18**(1):e14-e24

[59] Rostami A, Ma G, Wang T, Koehler AV, Hofmann A, Chang BCH, et al. Human toxocariasis – A look at a neglected disease through an epidemiological 'prism'. Infection, Genetics and Evolution. 2019;**74**:104002

[60] Fan C-K, Holland CV, Loxton K, Barghouth U. Cerebral Toxocariasis:

Silent progression to neurodegenerative disorders? Clinical Microbiology Reviews. 2015;**28**(3):663-686

[61] Meliou M, Mavridis IN, Pyrgelis E-S, Agapiou E. Toxocariasis of the nervous system. Acta Parasitologica. 2020;**65**(2):291-299

[62] Othman AA, Abdel-Aleem GA, Saied EM, Mayah WW, Elatrash AM. Biochemical and immunopathological changes in experimental neurotoxocariasis. Molecular and Biochemical Parasitology. 2010;**172**(1):1-8

[63] Sanchez SS, Garcia HH, Nicoletti A. Clinical and magnetic resonance imaging findings of Neurotoxocariasis. Frontiers in Neurology. 2018;**9**:53

[64] Arpino C, Gattinara GC, Piergili D, Curatolo P. Toxocara infection and epilepsy in children: A case-control study. Epilepsia. 1990;**31**(1):33-36

[65] Nicoletti A, Bartoloni A, Sofia V, Mantella A, Nsengiyumva G, Frescaline G, et al. Epilepsy and toxocariasis: A case-control study in Burundi. Epilepsia. 2007;**48**(5):894-899

[66] Akyol A, Bicerol B, Ertug S, Ertabaklar H, Kiylioglu N. Epilepsy and seropositivity rates of *Toxocara canis* and toxoplasma gondii. Seizure-European Journal of Epilepsy. 2007;**16**(3):233-237

[67] Winkler AS, Blocher J, Auer H, Gotwald T, Matuja W, Schmutzhard E. Anticysticercal and antitoxocaral antibodies in people with epilepsy in rural Tanzania. Transactions of the Royal Society of Tropical Medicine and Hygiene. 2008;**102**(10):1032-1038

[68] Birbeck GL. Seizures in rural Zambia. Epilepsia. 2000;**41**(3):277-281

[69] Mushi D, Hunter E, Mtuya C, Mshana G, Aris E, Walker R. Social-cultural aspects of epilepsy in Kilimanjaro region, Tanzania: Knowledge and experience among patients and carers. Epilepsy & Behavior. 2011;**20**(2):338-343

[70] Nsengiyumva G, Druet-Cabanac M, Nzisabira L, Preux PM, Vergnenegre A. Economic evaluation of epilepsy in Kiremba (Burundi): A case-control study. Epilepsia. 2004;**45**(6):673-677

[71] Ogunrin OA. Epilepsy in Nigeria-a review of etiology; epidemiology and management. Benin Journal of Postgraduate Medicine. 2006;**8**(1):27-51

[72] Osuntokun BO, Adeuja AO, Nottidge VA, Bademosi O, Olumide A, Ige O, et al. Prevalence of the epilepsies in Nigerian Africans: A community-based study. Epilepsia. 1987;**28**(3):272-279

[73] Osuntokun BO, Schoenberg BS, Nottidge VA, Adeuja A, Kale O, Adeyefa A, et al. Research protocol for measuring the prevalence of neurologic disorders in developing countries. Neuroepidemiology. 1982;**1**(3):143-153

[74] Brieger WR, Oshiname FO, Ososanya OO. Stigma associated with onchocercal skin disease among those affected near the Ofiki and Oyan Rivers in Western Nigeria. Social Science & Medicine. 1998;**47**(7):841-852

[75] Gbenou H. Contribution à l'étude de l'association onchocercose-épilepsie. Résultats préliminaires d'une enquête neuroépidémiologique à Agbogbomé commune de Paouignan, sous-préfecture de Dassa-Zoumé, au Bénin [MD Thesis]. Cotonou: Cotonou Univ Natl du; 1995

[76] Ae-Ngibise KA, Akpalu B, Ngugi A, Akpalu A, Agbokey F, Adjei P, et al. Prevalence and risk factors for active

convulsive epilepsy in Kintampo, Ghana. The Pan African Medical Journal. 2015;**21**:29

[77] Farnarier G, Diop S, Coulibaly B, Arborio S, Dabo A, Diakite M, et al. Onchocerciasis and epilepsy. Epidemiological survey in Mali. Medicine Tropical (Mars). 2000;**60**(2):151-155

[78] Siewe JFN, Ngarka L, Tatah G, Mengnjo MK, Nfor LN, Chokote ES, et al. Clinical presentations of onchocerciasis-associated epilepsy (OAE) in Cameroon. Epilepsy & Behavior. 2019;**90**:70-78

[79] Gerrits C. A west African epilepsy focus. Lancet. 1983;**1**(8320):358

[80] Goudsmit J, van der Waals FW, Gajdusek C. Epilepsy in the Gbawein and Wroughbarh clan of Grand Bassa County, Liberia: The endemic occurrence of 'See-ee' in the native population. Neuroepidemiology. 1983;**2**(1-2):24-34

[81] Kaudjhis P. Les agrégats de l'épilepsie de M'brou: approche électroclinique et étiologique. Medical Thesis. Abidjan, Côte-d'Ivoire: Université Nationale de Côte d'Ivoire; 1995

[82] Nitiema P, Carabin H, Hounton S, Praet N, Cowan LD, Ganaba R, et al. Prevalence case-control study of epilepsy in three Burkina Faso villages. Acta Neurologica Scandinavica. 2012;**126**(4):270-278

[83] Balogou AA, Doh A, Grunitzky KE. Neurological disorders and endemic goiter: Comparative analysis of 2 provinces in Togo. Bulletin de la Societe de Pathologie Exotique. 2001;**94**(5):406-410

[84] Coleman R, Loppy L, Walraven G. The treatment gap and primary health care for people with epilepsy in rural Gambia. Bulletin of the World Health Organization. 2002;**80**(5):378-383

[85] Ndoye NF, Sow AD, Diop AG, Sessouma B, Sene-Diouf F, Boissy L, et al. Prevalence of epilepsy its treatment gap and knowledge, attitude and practice of its population in sub-urban Senegal an ILAE/IBE/WHO study. Seizure. 2005;**14**(2):106-111

[86] De Toffol B. Epilepsies: étiologie, diagnostic, évolution, pronostic, traitement. La Revue du praticien (Paris). 1995;**45**(7):885-891

[87] Mbuba CK, Ngugi AK, Newton CR, Carter JA. The epilepsy treatment gap in developing countries: A systematic review of the magnitude, causes, and intervention strategies. Epilepsia. 2008;**49**(9):1491-1503

[88] Ascoli M, Ferlazzo E, Gasparini S, Mastroianni G, Citraro R, Roberti R, et al. Epidemiology and outcomes of status epilepticus. International Journal of General Medicine. 2021;**14**:2965-2973

[89] Meyer AC, Dua T, Ma J, Saxena S, Birbeck G. Global disparities in the epilepsy treatment gap: A systematic review. Bulletin of the World Health Organization. 2010;**88**(4):260-266

[90] Mattson RH, Cramer JA, Collins JF, Smith DB, Delgado-Escueta AV, Browne TR, et al. Comparison of carbamazepine, phenobarbital, phenytoin, and primidone in partial and secondarily generalized tonic-clonic seizures. The New England Journal of Medicine. 1985;**313**(3):145-151

[91] Richens A, Davidson DL, Cartlidge NE, Easter DJ. A multicentre comparative trial of sodium valproate and carbamazepine in adult onset epilepsy. Adult EPITEG collaborative group. Journal of Neurology, Neurosurgery, and Psychiatry. 1994;**57**(6):682-687

[92] Ogunniyi A, Osuntokun BO. Effectiveness of anticonvulsant therapy in the epilepsies in Nigerian Africans. East African Medical Journal. 1991;**68**(9):707-713

[93] Wilmshurst JM, Cross JH, Newton C, Kakooza AM, Wammanda RD, Mallewa M, et al. Children with epilepsy in Africa: Recommendations from the international child neurology association/African child neurology association workshop. Journal of Child Neurology. 2013;**28**(5):633-644

[94] Boussinesq M, Chippaux JP, Ernould JC, Quillevere D, Prodhon J. Effect of repeated treatments with Ivermectin on the incidence of onchocerciasis in northern Cameroon. American Journal of Tropical Medicine and Hygiene. 1995;**53**(1):63-67

[95] Boatin BA. The current state of the onchocerciasis control Programme in West Africa. Tropical Doctor. 2003;**33**(4):209-214

[96] Leveque C. The use of insecticides in the onchocerciasis control programme and aquatic monitoring in West Africa. Ecotoxicology and Climate. 1989;**317**:335

[97] Nimaga K, Desplats D, Doumbo O, Farnarier G. Treatment with phenobarbital and monitoring of epileptic patients in rural Mali. Bulletin of the World Health Organization. 2002;**80**:532-537

[98] Placencia M, Sander JWAS, Shorvon SD, Ellison RH, Cascante SM. Validation of a screening questionnaire for the detection of epileptic seizures in epidemiological studies. Brain. 1992;**115**(3):783-794

[99] Boling W, Means M, Fletcher A. Quality of life and stigma in epilepsy, perspectives from selected regions of Asia and sub-Saharan Africa. Brain Sciences. 2018;**8**(4):59

[100] Jacoby A. Felt versus enacted stigma: A concept revisited. Social Science & Medicine. 1994;**38**(2):269-274

[101] Cochrane J. Patient education: Lessons from epilepsy. Patient Education and Counseling. 1995;**26**(1-3):25-31

[102] Newton CR, Garcia HH. Epilepsy in poor regions of the world. The Lancet. 2012;**380**(9848):1193-1201

[103] Otte WM, van Diessen E, van Eijsden P, van der Maas F, Patsalos PN, Newton PN, et al. Counterfeit antiepileptic drugs threaten community services in Guinea-Bissau and Nigeria. The Lancet Neurology. 2015;**14**(11):1075-1076